Welcome to **_"Carb Cycling Diet Plan & Cookbook,"_** your comprehensive guide to harnessing the power of strategic carbohydrate consumption for optimal health, weight loss, and muscle building. Whether you're a seasoned athlete, a fitness enthusiast, or someone seeking a sustainable approach to healthy living, this book is designed to provide you with the knowledge, tools, and delicious recipes to achieve your goals.

Carb cycling is a dietary strategy that alternates between high-carb and low-carb days, tailored to match your physical activity levels. This method not only supports weight loss and muscle growth but also helps regulate hormones, enhance metabolic flexibility, and boost energy levels. By following the structured meal plans and exercise routines outlined in this book, you'll learn how to maximize your body's potential and achieve lasting results.

Inside, you'll find:

- **_60-Day Meal Plans:_** Carefully curated to take the guesswork out of meal preparation, these plans are designed to align with your fitness goals and keep your taste buds satisfied.

- **_110 Delicious Recipes:_** From hearty breakfasts and satisfying lunches to delectable dinners and guilt-free desserts, these recipes are crafted to ensure you enjoy every bite while staying on track.

- **_Effective Exercise Plans:_** Tailored workouts that complement your carb cycling regimen, designed to enhance your strength, endurance, and overall fitness.

- **_Expert Guidance:_** Insights into the science behind carb cycling, practical tips for meal prepping, and strategies for overcoming common challenges.

Embark on this journey with us and discover how carb cycling can transform your body and your life. With the right balance of nutrition and exercise, you'll unlock the keys to a healthier, fitter, and more vibrant you. Let's get started!

Dear Valued Customer,

*Thank you so much for purchasing **Carb Cycling Diet Plan & Cookbook: Recipes for Weight Loss, Muscle Building, Effective Exercise Plans with 60-Day Meal Plans and 110 Delicious Recipes.** We are thrilled to have you join our community of health enthusiasts!*

Your commitment to a healthier lifestyle is commendable, and we are confident that this book will be a valuable resource on your journey. Inside, you'll find a wealth of information, from detailed diet plans to tasty and nutritious recipes, all designed to help you achieve your fitness goals.

We hope you enjoy experimenting with the 60-day meal plans and trying out the 110 delicious recipes curated specifically to support your carb cycling regimen. Remember, consistency is key, and we're here to support you every step of the way.

If you have any questions or need further assistance, please don't hesitate to reach out. Your satisfaction is our top priority.

Happy cooking and best of luck on your health and fitness journey!

Warm regards,

Daisy Robinson

1. Grilled chicken breast with steamed broccoli

Ingredient:

- 4 boneless, skinless chicken breasts (about 4•6 oz each)
- 1 lb broccoli florets
- 1 tbsp olive oil
- Salt and pepper to taste

Instructions:

1. Preheat grill or grill pan to medium•high heat.

2. Brush the chicken breasts lightly with olive oil and season with salt and pepper.

3. Grill the chicken for 4•6 minutes per side, or until cooked through and no longer pink in the center. The internal temperature should reach 165°F.

4. While the chicken is grilling, steam the broccoli florets for 5•7 minutes until tender•crisp.

5. Serve the grilled chicken breast alongside the steamed broccoli.

This meal is a great option for a carb cycling diet plan as it is high in protein from the chicken, and low in carbs from the broccoli. The healthy fats from the olive oil also help to keep you feeling full and satisfied. Adjust the portion sizes as needed to fit your specific macronutrient requirements for the carb cycling phase.

2. Baked salmon with asparagus

Ingredient:

- 4 salmon fillets (4•6 oz each)
- 1 lb asparagus spears, trimmed
- 2 tbsp olive oil
- 1 tsp lemon zest
- Salt and pepper to taste

Instructions:

1. Preheat oven to 400°F.

2. Arrange the salmon fillets and asparagus spears on a large baking sheet. Drizzle with olive oil and sprinkle with lemon zest, salt, and pepper.

3. Bake for 12•15 minutes, or until the salmon is cooked through and flakes easily with a fork, and the asparagus is tender•crisp.

4. Serve the baked salmon immediately, with the roasted asparagus on the side.

This meal is a great option for a carb cycling diet plan as it is high in protein from the salmon, and low in carbs from the asparagus. The healthy fats from the olive oil and salmon also help to keep you feeling full and satisfied. Adjust the portion sizes as needed to fit your specific macronutrient requirements for the carb cycling phase.

3. Cauliflower rice stir-fry with tofu

Ingredient:

- 1 head of cauliflower, riced (about 4 cups riced cauliflower)
- 1 block of extra-firm tofu, cubed
- 2 tbsp sesame oil
- 2 cloves garlic, minced
- 1 inch fresh ginger, grated
- 1 cup sliced mushrooms
- 1 cup chopped bell peppers
- 2 cups chopped kale or spinach
- 2 tbsp low-sodium soy sauce or tamari
- Salt and pepper to taste

Instructions:

1. In a large skillet or wok, heat the sesame oil over medium-high heat.

2. Add the cubed tofu and sauté for 5-7 minutes, until lightly browned on all sides. Remove the tofu from the pan and set aside.

3. In the same pan, add the minced garlic and grated ginger. Sauté for 1 minute until fragrant.

4. Add the riced cauliflower, mushrooms, bell peppers, and kale/spinach. Stir-fry for 5-7 minutes, until the vegetables are tender-crisp.

5. Return the sautéed tofu to the pan and add the soy sauce. Toss everything together and season with salt and pepper to taste.

6. Serve the cauliflower rice stir-fry immediately.

This meal is a great option for a carb cycling diet plan as it is low in carbs from the cauliflower rice, high in protein from the tofu, and packed with nutrient-dense vegetables. Adjust the portion sizes as needed to fit your specific macronutrient requirements for the carb cycling phase.

4. Zucchini noodles (zoodles) with marinara sauce

Ingredient:

• 4 medium zucchinis, spiralized or julienned into noodles
• 1 tbsp olive oil
• 2 cloves garlic, minced
• 1 (28 oz) can crushed tomatoes
• 2 tbsp fresh basil, chopped
• Salt and pepper to taste

Instructions:

1. In a large skillet, heat the olive oil over medium heat. Add the minced garlic and sauté for 1•2 minutes until fragrant.

2. Add the spiralized or julienned zucchini noodles to the skillet. Sauté for 3•5 minutes, until the zucchini is tender but still has a slight bite.

3. Pour in the can of crushed tomatoes and stir to combine. Simmer for 5•7 minutes, allowing the flavors to meld.

4. Remove from heat and stir in the chopped fresh basil. Season with salt and pepper to taste.

5. Serve the zucchini noodles with the marinara sauce immediately.

This meal is a great option for a carb cycling diet plan as it is low in carbs from the zucchini noodles, and provides a good source of fiber and nutrients. The marinara sauce adds flavor without adding a significant amount of carbs. Adjust the portion sizes as needed to fit your specific macronutrient requirements for the carb cycling phase.

5. Turkey lettuce wraps with avocado

Ingredient:

- 1 lb ground turkey
- 1 tbsp olive oil
- 1 onion, diced
- 2 cloves garlic, minced
- 1 tbsp low•sodium soy sauce or tamari
- 1 tsp ground cumin
- 1 tsp chili powder
- Salt and pepper to taste
- 1 head of romaine or butter lettuce, leaves separated
- 1 avocado, sliced

Instructions:

1. In a large skillet, heat the olive oil over medium•high heat. Add the diced onion and sauté for 3•5 minutes until translucent.

2. Add the ground turkey, minced garlic, soy sauce, cumin, and chili powder. Cook, breaking up the turkey with a spatula, until the turkey is cooked through and no longer pink, about 7•10 minutes.

3. Season the turkey mixture with salt and pepper to taste.

4. To assemble the wraps, place a few spoonfuls of the turkey mixture into a lettuce leaf. Top with sliced avocado.

5. Serve the turkey lettuce wraps immediately.

This meal is a great option for a carb cycling diet plan as it is low in carbs from the lettuce wraps, high in protein from the turkey, and provides healthy fats from the avocado. Adjust the portion sizes as needed to fit your specific macronutrient requirements for the carb cycling phase.

6. Eggplant Parmesan (using almond flour for coating)

Ingredient:

- 2 medium eggplants, sliced into 1/2•inch thick rounds
- 1 cup almond flour
- 1 tsp dried oregano
- 1 tsp garlic powder
- 1/2 tsp salt
- 2 eggs, beaten
- 1 cup shredded mozzarella cheese
- 1/2 cup grated Parmesan cheese
- 1 (24 oz) jar marinara sauce

Instructions:

1. Preheat oven to 375°F. Line a baking sheet with parchment paper.

2. In a shallow bowl, mix together the almond flour, oregano, garlic powder, and salt.

3. Dip the eggplant slices into the beaten eggs, then coat them in the almond flour mixture, pressing gently to adhere.

4. Arrange the coated eggplant slices in a single layer on the prepared baking sheet.

5. Bake for 20•25 minutes, flipping halfway, until the eggplant is tender and the coating is golden brown.

6. Remove the eggplant from the oven and top each slice with a spoonful of marinara sauce, followed by the mozzarella and Parmesan cheeses.

7. Return the eggplant to the oven and bake for an additional 10•15 minutes, or until the cheese is melted and bubbly.

8. Serve the eggplant parmesan immediately.

This recipe is a great option for a carb cycling diet plan as it uses almond flour instead of traditional breadcrumbs, keeping the carb count low. The eggplant provides fiber, while the cheese and marinara sauce add protein and flavor. Adjust the portion sizes as needed to fit your specific macronutrient requirements.

7. Greek salad with feta cheese and olives

Ingredient:

- 6 cups chopped romaine lettuce
- 1 cup cherry tomatoes, halved
- 1/2 cup sliced cucumber
- 1/4 cup sliced red onion
- 1/4 cup pitted kalamata olives, halved
- 1/4 cup crumbled feta cheese
- 2 tbsp olive oil
- 1 tbsp red wine vinegar
- 1 tsp dried oregano
- Salt and pepper to taste

Instructions:

1. In a large salad bowl, combine the chopped romaine lettuce, cherry tomatoes, sliced cucumber, red onion, and kalamata olives.

2. Sprinkle the crumbled feta cheese over the top of the salad.

3. In a small bowl, whisk together the olive oil, red wine vinegar, and dried oregano. Season with salt and pepper to taste.

4. Drizzle the dressing over the salad and toss gently to coat.

5. Serve the Greek salad immediately.

This salad is a great option for a carb cycling diet plan as it is low in carbs, high in healthy fats from the olive oil and olives, and provides a good source of protein from the feta cheese. The vegetables also provide fiber and essential nutrients. Adjust the portion sizes as needed to fit your specific macronutrient requirements for the carb cycling phase.

8. Stir-fried shrimp with snow peas

Ingredient:

- 1 lb raw shrimp, peeled and deveined
- 2 tbsp sesame oil
- 2 cloves garlic, minced
- 1 inch fresh ginger, grated
- 1 cup snow peas, trimmed and halved diagonally
- 2 tbsp low•sodium soy sauce or tamari
- 1 tsp sesame seeds (optional)
- Salt and pepper to taste

Instructions:

1. In a large skillet or wok, heat the sesame oil over high heat.

2. Add the minced garlic and grated ginger. Sauté for 1 minute until fragrant.

3. Add the shrimp to the pan and stir•fry for 2•3 minutes, until the shrimp start to turn pink and curl.

4. Add the snow peas and continue to stir•fry for another 2•3 minutes, until the snow peas are tender•crisp.

5. Pour in the soy sauce and toss everything together to coat.

6. Remove from heat and sprinkle with sesame seeds, if using.

7. Season with salt and pepper to taste.

8. Serve the stir•fried shrimp and snow peas immediately.

This dish is a great option for a carb cycling diet plan as it is low in carbs, high in protein from the shrimp, and provides a good source of fiber from the snow peas. The healthy fats from the sesame oil also help to keep you feeling full and satisfied. Adjust the portion sizes as needed to fit your specific macronutrient requirements for the carb cycling phase.

9. Stuffed bell peppers with ground turkey and spinach

Ingredient:

• 4 bell peppers, halved and seeded
• 1 lb ground turkey
• 1 cup cooked spinach, chopped
• 1/2 cup diced onion
• 2 cloves garlic, minced
• 1 tsp dried oregano
• 1/2 tsp red pepper flakes (optional)
• Salt and pepper to taste
• 1/2 cup shredded mozzarella cheese

Instructions:

1. Preheat oven to 375°F.

2. In a large skillet, cook the ground turkey over medium•high heat, breaking it up with a spatula, until no longer pink, about 5•7 minutes.

3. Add the diced onion and minced garlic to the skillet. Sauté for 2•3 minutes until the onion is translucent.

4. Stir in the chopped spinach, dried oregano, and red pepper flakes (if using). Season with salt and pepper to taste.

5. Arrange the bell pepper halves in a baking dish. Spoon the turkey and spinach mixture evenly into the pepper halves.

6. Top each stuffed pepper with a sprinkle of shredded mozzarella cheese.

7. Bake for 20•25 minutes, or until the peppers are tender and the cheese is melted and bubbly.

8. Serve the stuffed bell peppers immediately.

This dish is a great option for a carb cycling diet plan as it is low in carbs, high in protein from the ground turkey, and provides a good source of fiber and nutrients from the bell peppers and spinach. Adjust the portion sizes as needed to fit your specific macronutrient requirements for the carb cycling phase.

10. Spinach and mushroom omelet

Ingredient:

- 3 eggs
- 1 cup fresh spinach, chopped
- 1/2 cup sliced mushrooms
- 1 tbsp olive oil
- Salt and pepper to taste

Instructions:

1. Heat the olive oil in a non•stick skillet over medium heat.

2. In a small bowl, whisk the eggs together until well combined.

3. Add the chopped spinach and sliced mushrooms to the skillet and sauté for 2•3 minutes until the vegetables are tender.

4. Pour the whisked eggs over the vegetables and let cook for 2•3 minutes, until the bottom is set.

5. Use a spatula to gently lift the edges of the omelet and tilt the pan to allow the uncooked egg to flow to the edges.

6. Once the omelet is mostly set, fold it in half and slide it onto a plate.

7. Season with salt and pepper to taste.

This omelet is high in protein from the eggs, and the spinach and mushrooms provide fiber and nutrients without adding many carbs. It's a great option for a carb cycling diet plan when you want a low•carb meal.

11. Chicken and vegetable skewers

Ingredient:

- 1 lb boneless, skinless chicken breasts, cut into 1•inch cubes
- 1 red bell pepper, cut into 1•inch pieces
- 1 zucchini, cut into 1•inch pieces
- 1 red onion, cut into 1•inch pieces
- 2 tbsp olive oil
- 1 tsp dried oregano
- 1 tsp garlic powder
- Salt and pepper to taste

Instructions:

1. Preheat your grill or grill pan to medium•high heat.

2. In a large bowl, combine the chicken, bell pepper, zucchini, and onion. Drizzle with the olive oil and sprinkle with the oregano, garlic powder, salt, and pepper. Toss to coat the ingredients evenly.

3. Thread the chicken and vegetables onto skewers, alternating the ingredients.

4. Grill the skewers for 12•15 minutes, turning occasionally, until the chicken is cooked through and the vegetables are tender.

5. Serve the chicken and vegetable skewers immediately.

This dish is a great option for a carb cycling diet plan because it's high in protein from the chicken and low in carbs from the vegetables. The grilled vegetables also provide fiber and nutrients without adding many carbs. You can adjust the portion sizes to fit your specific carb cycling plan.

12. Baked cod with a side of mixed greens

Ingredient:

- 4 (6 oz) cod fillets
- 2 tbsp olive oil
- 1 tsp lemon zest
- 1 tbsp lemon juice
- 1 tsp dried parsley
- Salt and pepper to taste
- 4 cups mixed greens (such as spinach, arugula, and kale)
- 1 tbsp balsamic vinegar
- 1 tsp Dijon mustard

Instructions:

1. Preheat your oven to 400°F (200°C).

2. In a small bowl, mix together the olive oil, lemon zest, lemon juice, and dried parsley. Season the cod fillets with salt and pepper, then brush the top of each fillet with the lemon•herb mixture.

3. Place the cod fillets on a baking sheet lined with parchment paper. Bake for 12•15 minutes, or until the cod is opaque and flakes easily with a fork.

4. In a large salad bowl, combine the mixed greens. In a small bowl, whisk together the balsamic vinegar and Dijon mustard. Drizzle the vinaigrette over the greens and toss to coat.

5. Serve the baked cod fillets with the mixed greens salad.

This dish is a great option for a carb cycling diet plan because the cod is a lean protein source, and the mixed greens provide fiber and nutrients without adding many carbs. The balsamic vinaigrette dressing adds flavor without adding a significant amount of carbs.

13. Cabbage rolls with ground beef

Ingredient:

- 1 medium head of green cabbage
- 1 lb ground beef
- 1 onion, finely chopped
- 2 cloves garlic, minced
- 1 cup cooked cauliflower rice (or riced broccoli)
- 1 tsp dried oregano
- 1 tsp dried basil
- Salt and pepper to taste
- 1 (15 oz) can tomato sauce

Instructions:

1. Bring a large pot of water to a boil. Core the cabbage and carefully place it in the boiling water. Cook for 5•7 minutes, or until the outer leaves are tender and pliable. Remove the cabbage from the water and let cool.

2. In a large bowl, combine the ground beef, onion, garlic, cauliflower rice, oregano, basil, salt, and pepper. Mix well.

3. Carefully peel the outer leaves off the cabbage, one at a time, and place about 2•3 tablespoons of the beef mixture in the center of each leaf. Fold the sides of the leaf over the filling and roll up tightly.

4. Place the cabbage rolls seam•side down in a baking dish. Pour the tomato sauce over the top.

5. Bake at 375°F (190°C) for 45•60 minutes, or until the cabbage rolls are heated through and the beef is cooked.

This dish is a great option for a carb cycling diet plan because the cabbage leaves replace traditional rice or pasta, and the ground beef provides a good source of protein. The cauliflower rice adds fiber and nutrients without adding many carbs.

14. Caprese salad with mozzarella, tomatoes, and basil

Ingredient:

- 8 oz fresh mozzarella cheese, sliced
- 2 cups cherry or grape tomatoes, halved
- 1/4 cup fresh basil leaves, chopped
- 2 tbsp olive oil
- 1 tbsp balsamic vinegar
- Salt and pepper to taste

Instructions:

1. Arrange the sliced mozzarella cheese and halved tomatoes on a serving platter or plate.

2. Sprinkle the chopped fresh basil leaves over the top.

3. Drizzle the olive oil and balsamic vinegar over the salad.

4. Season with salt and pepper to taste.

This Caprese salad is a great option for a carb cycling diet plan because it's low in carbs and high in healthy fats and protein from the mozzarella cheese. The tomatoes and basil provide additional nutrients without adding many carbs.

You can adjust the portion sizes to fit your specific carb cycling plan. For example, you could serve this as a side salad or a light main dish, depending on your daily carb intake goals.

The simple dressing of olive oil and balsamic vinegar adds flavor without adding any additional carbs. This Caprese salad is a refreshing and nutritious option for a carb cycling diet.

15. Grilled steak with a side of roasted Brussels sprouts

Ingredient:

Steak:
- 1 lb flank steak or sirloin steak
- 1 tbsp olive oil
- 1 tsp garlic powder
- 1 tsp onion powder
- Salt and pepper to taste

Brussels Sprouts:
- 1 lb Brussels sprouts, trimmed and halved
- 2 tbsp olive oil
- 1 tsp garlic powder
- Salt and pepper to taste

Instructions:

Steak:
1. Preheat your grill or grill pan to high heat.
2. Rub the steak with the olive oil, garlic powder, onion powder, salt, and pepper.
3. Grill the steak for 3•5 minutes per side, or until it reaches your desired level of doneness.
4. Let the steak rest for 5 minutes before slicing.

Brussels Sprouts:
1. Preheat your oven to 400°F (200°C).
2. In a large bowl, toss the Brussels sprouts with the olive oil, garlic powder, salt, and pepper.
3. Spread the Brussels sprouts in a single layer on a baking sheet.
4. Roast for 20•25 minutes, or until the Brussels sprouts are tender and lightly browned.

Serve the grilled steak with the roasted Brussels sprouts. This meal is a great option for a carb cycling diet plan because the steak provides a lean protein source, and the Brussels sprouts are a low•carb vegetable that is high in fiber and nutrients.

You can adjust the portion sizes of the steak and Brussels sprouts to fit your specific carb cycling plan.

16. Ratatouille (vegetable stew)

Ingredient:

- 1 medium eggplant, diced
- 1 medium zucchini, diced
- 1 medium yellow squash, diced
- 1 red bell pepper, diced
- 1 onion, diced
- 3 cloves garlic, minced
- 2 tbsp olive oil
- 1 (14 oz) can diced tomatoes
- 2 tbsp tomato paste
- 1 tsp dried thyme
- 1 tsp dried oregano
- Salt and pepper to taste
- 2 tbsp chopped fresh basil (optional)

Instructions:

1. In a large skillet or Dutch oven, heat the olive oil over medium heat.

2. Add the diced eggplant, zucchini, yellow squash, bell pepper, onion, and garlic. Sauté for 8•10 minutes, or until the vegetables are starting to soften.

3. Add the diced tomatoes, tomato paste, thyme, oregano, salt, and pepper. Stir to combine.

4. Reduce the heat to low, cover the pot, and simmer for 20•25 minutes, or until the vegetables are very tender.

5. Remove from heat and stir in the chopped fresh basil, if using.

6. Serve the ratatouille warm, as a main dish or side.

This ratatouille is a great option for a carb cycling diet plan because it's packed with low•carb vegetables like eggplant, zucchini, and bell pepper. The tomatoes and tomato paste provide some carbs, but the overall carb content is still relatively low. You can adjust the portion sizes to fit your specific carb cycling plan.

17. Egg drop soup with chicken and vegetables

Ingredient:

- 4 cups low•sodium chicken broth
- 1 boneless, skinless chicken breast, diced
- 1 cup sliced mushrooms
- 1 cup chopped spinach
- 2 eggs, lightly beaten
- 1 tsp sesame oil
- 1 tsp low•sodium soy sauce
- Salt and pepper to taste

Instructions:

1. In a medium saucepan, bring the chicken broth to a simmer over medium heat.

2. Add the diced chicken, mushrooms, and spinach to the broth. Simmer for 5•7 minutes, or until the chicken is cooked through and the vegetables are tender.

3. Slowly drizzle the beaten eggs into the simmering broth, stirring gently to create ribbons of egg.

4. Remove the soup from heat and stir in the sesame oil and soy sauce.

5. Season with salt and pepper to taste.

6. Serve the egg drop soup hot.

This egg drop soup is a great option for a carb cycling diet plan because it's low in carbs and high in protein from the chicken and eggs. The vegetables provide fiber and nutrients without adding many carbs.

The broth•based soup is also a light and hydrating option, which can be beneficial during a carb cycling plan. You can adjust the portion sizes to fit your specific carb intake goals for the day.

18. Spaghetti squash with pesto sauce

Ingredient:

- 1 medium spaghetti squash
- 2 cups fresh basil leaves
- 1/4 cup pine nuts
- 2 cloves garlic
- 1/4 cup grated Parmesan cheese
- 2 tbsp olive oil
- Salt and pepper to taste

Instructions:

1. Preheat your oven to 400°F (200°C).

2. Cut the spaghetti squash in half lengthwise and scoop out the seeds. Place the squash halves cut•side down on a baking sheet lined with parchment paper.

3. Bake the spaghetti squash for 30•40 minutes, or until it's tender and easily shreds with a fork.

4. While the squash is baking, make the pesto sauce. In a food processor, combine the fresh basil leaves, pine nuts, garlic, Parmesan cheese, and olive oil. Pulse until a smooth pesto forms. Season with salt and pepper to taste.

5. Once the spaghetti squash is cooked, use a fork to shred the flesh into spaghetti•like strands.

6. Serve the spaghetti squash strands warm, topped with the pesto sauce.

This spaghetti squash dish is a great option for a carb cycling diet plan because the squash provides a low•carb alternative to traditional pasta. The pesto sauce is high in healthy fats from the olive oil and pine nuts, and the Parmesan cheese adds protein without many carbs.

You can adjust the portion sizes of the spaghetti squash and pesto to fit your specific carb cycling plan. This dish is a delicious and nutritious way to enjoy a pasta•like meal while staying on track with your carb cycling goals.

19. Seared tuna steak with a side of steamed green beans

Ingredient:

Tuna Steak:
- 4 (6 oz) tuna steaks
- 1 tbsp olive oil
- 1 tsp garlic powder
- 1 tsp onion powder
- Salt and pepper to taste

Green Beans:
- 1 lb fresh green beans, trimmed
- 1 tbsp butter
- Salt and pepper to taste

Instructions:

Tuna Steak:
1. Pat the tuna steaks dry with paper towels and season both sides with the garlic powder, onion powder, salt, and pepper.

2. Heat the olive oil in a large skillet over high heat.

3. Sear the tuna steaks for 2•3 minutes per side, or until the outside is lightly browned but the center is still pink.

4. Remove the tuna steaks from the heat and let them rest for 5 minutes before serving.

Green Beans:
1. Fill a medium saucepan with 1•2 inches of water and bring to a boil.

2. Add the trimmed green beans and steam for 5•7 minutes, or until the beans are tender•crisp.

3. Drain the green beans and toss with the butter. Season with salt and pepper to taste.

Serve the seared tuna steaks with the steamed green beans. This meal is a great option for a carb cycling diet plan because the tuna provides a lean protein source, and the green beans are a low•carb vegetable that is high in fiber and nutrients.

You can adjust the portion sizes of the tuna and green beans to fit your specific carb cycling plan.

20. Portobello mushroom burgers with lettuce buns

Ingredient:

- 4 large portobello mushroom caps, stems removed
- 2 tbsp olive oil
- 1 tsp garlic powder
- 1 tsp onion powder
- Salt and pepper to taste
- 4 large lettuce leaves (such as romaine or butter lettuce)
- Desired toppings (e.g., tomato slices, avocado, cheese, etc.)

Instructions:

1. Preheat your grill or grill pan to medium•high heat.

2. Brush the portobello mushroom caps with the olive oil and season with the garlic powder, onion powder, salt, and pepper.

3. Grill the mushroom caps for 4•5 minutes per side, or until they are tender and slightly charred.

4. Place each grilled mushroom cap on a large lettuce leaf to use as the "bun."

5. Top the mushroom burgers with your desired toppings.

This portobello mushroom burger is a great option for a carb cycling diet plan because the mushroom caps replace the traditional bun, which is typically high in carbs. The lettuce leaves also provide a low•carb alternative to a traditional burger bun.

You can customize the toppings to your liking, but be mindful of the carb content of any additional ingredients. Avocado, tomatoes, and cheese are all good low•carb options.

Serve these portobello mushroom burgers with a side salad or other low•carb vegetable for a complete and satisfying meal that fits within your carb cycling plan.

21. Tofu stir-fry with bell peppers and snap peas

Ingredient:

- 1 block (14 oz) extra-firm tofu, cubed
- 2 tbsp sesame oil
- 1 red bell pepper, sliced
- 1 yellow bell pepper, sliced
- 1 cup snap peas, trimmed
- 2 cloves garlic, minced
- 1 tbsp grated fresh ginger
- 2 tbsp low-sodium soy sauce
- 1 tsp rice vinegar
- Salt and pepper to taste
- Chopped green onions for garnish (optional)

Instructions:

1. Heat the sesame oil in a large skillet or wok over medium-high heat.

2. Add the cubed tofu and cook, stirring occasionally, until lightly browned on all sides, about 5-7 minutes. Transfer the tofu to a plate and set aside.

3. Add the sliced bell peppers and snap peas to the skillet. Stir-fry for 3-4 minutes, until the vegetables are crisp-tender.

4. Add the minced garlic and grated ginger to the skillet. Cook for 1 minute, stirring constantly, until fragrant.

5. Return the cooked tofu to the skillet. Add the soy sauce and rice vinegar. Toss everything together and cook for an additional 2-3 minutes, until the sauce has thickened slightly.

6. Season with salt and pepper to taste. Serve the tofu stir-fry hot, garnished with chopped green onions if desired.

This tofu stir-fry is a great option for a carb cycling diet plan because it's low in carbs and high in protein from the tofu. The bell peppers and snap peas provide fiber and nutrients without adding many carbs.

You can adjust the portion sizes to fit your specific carb cycling plan. Serve this stir-fry over a bed of cauliflower rice or with a side of steamed broccoli for an even more low-carb meal.

22. Greek yogurt with berries and nuts

Ingredient:

- 1 cup plain Greek yogurt
- 1/2 cup mixed berries (such as blueberries, raspberries, and/or blackberries)
- 2 tbsp chopped nuts (such as almonds, walnuts, or pecans)
- 1 tsp honey (optional)

Instructions:

1. In a bowl, place the Greek yogurt.

2. Top the yogurt with the mixed berries.

3. Sprinkle the chopped nuts over the berries.

4. If desired, drizzle the honey over the top.

This Greek yogurt with berries and nuts is a great option for a carb cycling diet plan for a few reasons:

1. Greek yogurt is high in protein and low in carbs, making it a great choice for a carb cycling meal or snack.

2. Berries are a low•glycemic fruit, meaning they are lower in carbs and won't spike your blood sugar as much as other fruits.

3. Nuts provide healthy fats and a bit of protein, which can help keep you feeling full and satisfied.

The honey is optional, as it does add a small amount of carbs, but you can omit it or use just a small drizzle if you want to keep the carb count even lower.

You can adjust the portion sizes of the yogurt, berries, and nuts to fit your specific carb cycling plan. This makes for a delicious and nutritious snack or light meal.

23. Shrimp ceviche

Ingredient:

- 1 lb raw shrimp, peeled, deveined, and chopped
- 1 cup fresh lime juice (about 6•8 limes)
- 1 cup diced tomatoes
- 1/2 cup diced red onion
- 1/2 cup diced cucumber
- 1/4 cup chopped cilantro
- 1 jalapeño, seeded and minced (optional)
- Salt and pepper to taste

Instructions:

1. In a large non•reactive bowl (glass or stainless steel), combine the chopped shrimp and lime juice. Cover and refrigerate for 30•60 minutes, or until the shrimp is opaque and "cooked" through the acid in the lime juice.

2. Drain any excess lime juice from the shrimp.

3. Add the diced tomatoes, red onion, cucumber, cilantro, and jalapeño (if using). Stir to combine.

4. Season with salt and pepper to taste.

5. Serve the shrimp ceviche chilled, with lettuce leaves or endive leaves for scooping, if desired.

This shrimp ceviche is a great option for a carb cycling diet plan because it's low in carbs and high in protein from the shrimp. The fresh vegetables provide fiber and nutrients without adding many carbs.

The lime juice "cooks" the shrimp without the need for heat, making this a refreshing and light dish. You can adjust the portion sizes to fit your specific carb cycling plan.

Serve this shrimp ceviche as a main dish or as a healthy appetizer. It's a delicious and nutritious way to enjoy seafood while following a carb cycling diet.

24. Chicken lettuce wraps with Asian-inspired sauce

Ingredient:

Chicken Filling:
- 1 lb ground chicken or finely chopped chicken breast
- 1 tbsp sesame oil
- 2 cloves garlic, minced
- 1 tbsp grated fresh ginger
- 2 tbsp low-sodium soy sauce
- 1 tsp rice vinegar
- 1/4 tsp red pepper flakes (optional)
- Salt and pepper to taste

Sauce:
- 2 tbsp low-sodium soy sauce
- 1 tbsp rice vinegar
- 1 tsp sesame oil
- 1 tsp honey
- 1 tsp Dijon mustard
- 1 clove garlic, minced
- Salt and pepper to taste

Wraps:
- 8-10 large lettuce leaves (such as romaine or butter lettuce)
- Chopped green onions, for garnish

Instructions:

1. In a large skillet or wok, heat the sesame oil over medium-high heat. Add the ground chicken, garlic, and ginger. Cook, breaking up the chicken with a spatula, until the chicken is cooked through, about 5-7 minutes.

2. Stir in the soy sauce, rice vinegar, red pepper flakes (if using), and season with salt and pepper.

3. In a small bowl, whisk together all the sauce ingredients.

4. To assemble, place a spoonful of the chicken mixture into the center of a lettuce leaf. Drizzle with the Asian-inspired sauce and top with chopped green onions. Serve the chicken lettuce wraps immediately.

This dish is a great option for a carb cycling diet plan because the lettuce leaves replace traditional high-carb wraps or buns, and the chicken provides a lean protein source. The Asian-inspired sauce adds flavor without adding many carbs.

You can adjust the portion sizes of the chicken filling and sauce to fit your specific carb cycling plan. Serve this as a main dish or as a low-carb appetizer.

25. Stuffed mushrooms with sausage and cheese

Ingredient:
- 12 large mushrooms, stems removed and finely chopped
- 1/2 lb ground Italian sausage, casings removed
- 1/4 cup grated Parmesan cheese
- 2 oz cream cheese, softened
- 1 clove garlic, minced
- 1 tbsp chopped fresh parsley
- Salt and pepper to taste

Instructions:
1. Preheat your oven to 375°F (190°C).

2. In a skillet over medium heat, cook the ground sausage until browned and crumbled, about 5•7 minutes. Drain any excess fat.

3. In a medium bowl, combine the chopped mushroom stems, cooked sausage, Parmesan cheese, cream cheese, garlic, and parsley. Season with salt and pepper.

4. Stuff the mushroom caps with the sausage mixture, packing it in tightly.

5. Arrange the stuffed mushrooms on a baking sheet lined with parchment paper.

6. Bake for 15•20 minutes, or until the mushrooms are tender and the filling is hot and bubbly. Serve the stuffed mushrooms warm.

These stuffed mushrooms are a great option for a carb cycling diet plan because they are low in carbs and high in protein and healthy fats. The sausage and cheese provide the bulk of the filling, while the mushroom caps act as a low•carb vessel.

You can adjust the portion sizes to fit your specific carb cycling plan. These stuffed mushrooms can be served as an appetizer or a light main dish, depending on your daily carb intake goals.

The combination of savory sausage, creamy cheese, and earthy mushrooms makes these stuffed mushrooms a delicious and satisfying option for a carb cycling diet.

26. Quinoa and black bean salad

Ingredient:

- 1 cup cooked quinoa, cooled
- 1 (15 oz) can black beans, rinsed and drained
- 1 cup diced cucumber
- 1 cup diced tomatoes
- 1/2 cup diced red onion
- 1/4 cup chopped fresh cilantro
- 2 tbsp olive oil
- 1 tbsp lime juice
- 1 tsp ground cumin
- Salt and pepper to taste

Instructions:

1. In a large bowl, combine the cooked quinoa, black beans, cucumber, tomatoes, red onion, and cilantro.

2. In a small bowl, whisk together the olive oil, lime juice, and cumin. Season with salt and pepper.

3. Pour the dressing over the quinoa and bean mixture and toss gently to coat.

4. Refrigerate the salad for at least 30 minutes to allow the flavors to meld.

5. Serve chilled or at room temperature.

This quinoa and black bean salad is a great option for a carb cycling diet plan for a few reasons:

1. Quinoa is a high•protein, gluten•free grain that is relatively low in carbs compared to other grains.
2. Black beans provide fiber, protein, and complex carbs, making them a good choice for a carb cycling plan.
3. The vegetables, herbs, and simple dressing add flavor and nutrients without significantly increasing the carb content.

You can adjust the portion sizes to fit your specific carb cycling plan. This salad can be served as a main dish or a side, depending on your daily carb intake goals.

The combination of protein, fiber, and complex carbs from the quinoa and black beans makes this a filling and nutritious option for a carb cycling diet.

27. Grilled chicken Caesar salad with croutons

Ingredient:

Salad:
- 4 boneless, skinless chicken breasts
- 1 romaine lettuce heart, chopped
- 1/2 cup shredded Parmesan cheese
- 2 tbsp low•carb croutons (optional)

Dressing:
- 1/4 cup olive oil
- 2 tbsp lemon juice
- 1 tbsp Dijon mustard
- 1 clove garlic, minced
- 1 tsp Worcestershire sauce
- Salt and pepper to taste

Instructions:

1. Preheat your grill or grill pan to medium•high heat.

2. Season the chicken breasts with salt and pepper.

3. Grill the chicken for 5•7 minutes per side, or until cooked through. Let the chicken rest for 5 minutes, then slice or chop it.

4. In a small bowl, whisk together the olive oil, lemon juice, Dijon mustard, garlic, and Worcestershire sauce. Season the dressing with salt and pepper to taste.

5. In a large salad bowl, combine the chopped romaine lettuce, grilled chicken, Parmesan cheese, and croutons (if using).

6. Drizzle the Caesar dressing over the salad and toss to coat. Serve the grilled chicken Caesar salad immediately.

This grilled chicken Caesar salad is a great option for a carb cycling diet plan because it's low in carbs and high in protein from the chicken. The romaine lettuce and Parmesan cheese provide nutrients without adding many carbs.

The optional croutons can be included in moderation, as they do add a small amount of carbs. You can also omit the croutons entirely to keep the carb count even lower.

Adjust the portion sizes of the chicken, lettuce, and dressing to fit your specific carb cycling plan. This salad makes for a satisfying and nutritious meal that fits well within a carb cycling diet.

28. Turkey chili with beans

Ingredient:

- 1 lb ground turkey
- 1 onion, diced
- 3 cloves garlic, minced
- 1 jalapeño, seeded and diced (optional)
- 2 tbsp chili powder
- 1 tsp ground cumin
- 1 tsp dried oregano
- 1 tsp paprika
- 1/2 tsp cayenne pepper (optional)
- 1 (15 oz) can diced tomatoes
- 1 (15 oz) can black beans, rinsed and drained
- 1 (15 oz) can kidney beans, rinsed and drained
- Salt and pepper to taste
- Chopped cilantro for garnish (optional)

Instructions:

1. In a large pot or Dutch oven, cook the ground turkey over medium•high heat, breaking it up with a wooden spoon, until browned, about 5•7 minutes.

2. Add the diced onion, minced garlic, and diced jalapeño (if using). Cook for 2•3 minutes, until the vegetables are softened.

3. Stir in the chili powder, cumin, oregano, paprika, and cayenne pepper (if using). Cook for 1 minute to toast the spices.

4. Add the diced tomatoes, black beans, and kidney beans. Stir to combine.

5. Bring the chili to a simmer and let it cook for 20•25 minutes, stirring occasionally, until the flavors have melded and the chili has thickened.

6. Season with salt and pepper to taste. Serve the turkey chili hot, garnished with chopped cilantro if desired.

This turkey chili with beans is a great option for a carb cycling diet plan because it's high in protein from the turkey and beans, and the beans provide fiber and complex carbs without too many net carbs.

You can adjust the portion sizes to fit your specific carb cycling plan. Serve this chili on its own or with a side of roasted vegetables for a complete and satisfying meal.

The spices and beans make this a flavorful and filling dish that fits well within a carb cycling diet.

29. Baked sweet potato with cottage cheese

Ingredient:

- 1 medium sweet potato
- 1/2 cup low•fat cottage cheese
- 1 tbsp chopped fresh chives (optional)
- Salt and pepper to taste

Instructions:

1. Preheat your oven to 400°F (200°C).

2. Wash the sweet potato and prick it several times with a fork.

3. Bake the sweet potato directly on the oven rack for 45•60 minutes, or until it's tender when pierced with a fork.

4. Remove the sweet potato from the oven and let it cool for 5 minutes.

5. Cut the sweet potato in half lengthwise and top each half with 1/4 cup of the cottage cheese.

6. Sprinkle the chopped chives (if using) over the top and season with salt and pepper to taste.

This baked sweet potato with cottage cheese is a great option for a carb cycling diet plan for a few reasons:

1. Sweet potatoes are a complex carbohydrate that is lower on the glycemic index compared to regular potatoes, making them a better choice for carb cycling.

2. Cottage cheese is a high•protein, low•carb dairy product that can help balance the carbs from the sweet potato.

3. The combination of the sweet potato and cottage cheese provides a satisfying and nutrient•dense meal or snack.

You can adjust the portion size of the sweet potato and cottage cheese to fit your specific carb cycling plan. This dish can be enjoyed as a main meal or a side dish, depending on your daily carb intake goals.

The optional chives add a fresh flavor, but you can omit them if desired. This baked sweet potato with cottage cheese is a simple and delicious option for a carb cycling diet.

30. Lentil soup with vegetables

Ingredient:

- 1 cup dry brown or green lentils, rinsed
- 4 cups low•sodium chicken or vegetable broth
- 1 tbsp olive oil
- 1 onion, diced
- 2 carrots, peeled and diced
- 2 celery stalks, diced
- 3 cloves garlic, minced
- 1 tsp dried thyme
- 1 tsp dried oregano
- Salt and pepper to taste
- Chopped parsley for garnish (optional)

Instructions:

1. In a large pot, combine the rinsed lentils and broth. Bring to a boil over high heat.

2. Reduce the heat to medium•low, cover, and simmer for 15•20 minutes, or until the lentils are tender.

3. In a separate skillet, heat the olive oil over medium heat. Add the diced onion, carrots, and celery. Sauté for 5•7 minutes, until the vegetables are softened.

4. Add the minced garlic, thyme, and oregano to the skillet. Cook for 1 minute, until fragrant.

5. Transfer the sautéed vegetables to the pot with the cooked lentils. Stir to combine.

6. Simmer the lentil soup for an additional 10•15 minutes, allowing the flavors to meld. Season the soup with salt and pepper to taste. Serve the lentil soup hot, garnished with chopped parsley if desired.

This lentil soup is a great option for a carb cycling diet plan because lentils are a low•glycemic, high•fiber legume that provides complex carbs and protein. The vegetables add fiber and nutrients without significantly increasing the carb content.

You can adjust the portion sizes to fit your specific carb cycling plan. This lentil soup can be served as a main dish or a side, depending on your daily carb intake goals.

The combination of the hearty lentils, flavorful vegetables, and savory spices makes this a satisfying and nutritious option for a carb cycling diet.

31. Beef and vegetable stir-fry with rice noodles

Ingredient:

- 8 oz rice noodles
- 1 lb flank steak, thinly sliced
- 2 tbsp sesame oil, divided
- 2 cloves garlic, minced
- 1 tbsp grated fresh ginger
- 1 red bell pepper, sliced
- 1 cup broccoli florets
- 1 cup snow peas
- 2 tbsp low•sodium soy sauce
- 1 tsp rice vinegar
- Salt and pepper to taste
- Chopped green onions for garnish (optional)

Instructions:

1. Prepare the rice noodles according to package instructions. Drain and set aside.

2. In a large skillet or wok, heat 1 tbsp of the sesame oil over high heat.

3. Add the sliced beef and stir•fry for 2•3 minutes, until browned. Transfer the beef to a plate and set aside.

4. Add the remaining 1 tbsp of sesame oil to the skillet. Add the minced garlic and grated ginger. Stir•fry for 1 minute until fragrant.

5. Add the sliced bell pepper, broccoli florets, and snow peas. Stir•fry for 3•4 minutes, until the vegetables are crisp•tender.

6. Return the cooked beef to the skillet. Add the cooked rice noodles, soy sauce, and rice vinegar. Toss everything together until well combined and heated through.

7. Season the stir•fry with salt and pepper to taste. Serve the beef and vegetable stir•fry with rice noodles, garnished with chopped green onions if desired.

This beef and vegetable stir•fry with rice noodles is a great option for a carb cycling diet plan. The rice noodles provide a lower•carb alternative to traditional pasta or rice, while the beef and vegetables offer a balance of protein, fiber, and nutrients.

You can adjust the portion sizes of the noodles, beef, and vegetables to fit your specific carb cycling plan. This dish is a flavorful and satisfying way to enjoy a stir•fry while staying on track with your carb cycling goals.

32. Whole grain pasta with marinara sauce

Ingredient:

- 2 tbsp tomato paste
- 1 tsp dried oregano
- 1 tsp dried basil
- Salt and pepper to taste
- Grated Parmesan cheese for serving (optional)

- 8 oz whole grain pasta (such as whole wheat or chickpea pasta)
- 1 tbsp olive oil
- 1 onion, diced
- 3 cloves garlic, minced
- 1 (28 oz) can crushed tomatoes

Instructions:

1. Bring a large pot of salted water to a boil. Cook the whole grain pasta according to the package instructions, until al dente. Drain and set aside.

2. In a large skillet, heat the olive oil over medium heat. Add the diced onion and sauté for 3•4 minutes, until translucent.

3. Add the minced garlic to the skillet and cook for 1 minute, until fragrant.

4. Pour in the crushed tomatoes and tomato paste. Stir in the dried oregano and basil. Season with salt and pepper to taste.

5. Simmer the marinara sauce for 10•15 minutes, stirring occasionally, to allow the flavors to meld.

6. Add the cooked whole grain pasta to the marinara sauce and toss to coat.

7. Serve the whole grain pasta with marinara sauce, topped with grated Parmesan cheese if desired.

This whole grain pasta with marinara sauce is a great option for a carb cycling diet plan for a few reasons:

1. Whole grain pasta is a complex carbohydrate that is higher in fiber and nutrients compared to refined pasta.

2. The marinara sauce is low in carbs and provides a good source of lycopene and other antioxidants. You can control the portion size of the pasta to fit your specific carb cycling plan.

Adjust the serving size of the pasta to align with your daily carb intake goals. Pair this dish with a side salad or roasted vegetables for a complete and balanced meal.

33. Grilled pork tenderloin with roasted potatoes

Ingredient:

Pork Tenderloin:
- 1 lb pork tenderloin
- 1 tbsp olive oil
- 1 tsp garlic powder
- 1 tsp onion powder
- Salt and pepper to taste

Roasted Potatoes:
- 1 lb baby potatoes, halved
- 1 tbsp olive oil
- 1 tsp dried rosemary
- Salt and pepper to taste

Instructions:

Pork Tenderloin:
1. Preheat your grill or grill pan to medium•high heat.
2. Rub the pork tenderloin with the olive oil, garlic powder, onion powder, salt, and pepper.
3. Grill the pork for 12•15 minutes, turning occasionally, until it reaches an internal temperature of 145°F (63°C).
4. Let the pork rest for 5 minutes before slicing.

Roasted Potatoes:
1. Preheat your oven to 400°F (200°C).
2. In a large bowl, toss the halved baby potatoes with the olive oil, dried rosemary, salt, and pepper.
3. Spread the potatoes in a single layer on a baking sheet.
4. Roast the potatoes for 20•25 minutes, or until they are tender and lightly browned.

Serve the grilled pork tenderloin with the roasted potatoes. This meal is a great option for a carb cycling diet plan because the pork provides a lean protein source, and the potatoes are a complex carbohydrate that is lower on the glycemic index compared to other starchy foods.

You can adjust the portion sizes of the pork and potatoes to fit your specific carb cycling plan. This dish is a delicious and satisfying way to enjoy a balanced meal while following a carb cycling diet.

34. Teriyaki chicken with brown rice

Ingredient:

Teriyaki Chicken:
- 1 lb boneless, skinless chicken breasts, cut into 1•inch pieces
- 2 tbsp low•sodium soy sauce
- 1 tbsp rice vinegar
- 1 tbsp honey
- 1 tsp sesame oil
- 2 cloves garlic, minced
- 1 tsp grated fresh ginger

Brown Rice:
- 1 cup uncooked brown rice
- 2 cups low•sodium chicken broth

Instructions:

Teriyaki Chicken:

1. In a large resealable bag or bowl, combine the chicken, soy sauce, rice vinegar, honey, sesame oil, garlic, and ginger. Toss to coat the chicken. Cover and marinate in the refrigerator for 30 minutes to 1 hour.
2. Heat a large skillet or wok over medium•high heat. Add the marinated chicken and cook for 6•8 minutes, stirring occasionally, until the chicken is cooked through and no longer pink.

Brown Rice:

1. In a medium saucepan, combine the brown rice and chicken broth. Bring to a boil over high heat.
2. Once boiling, reduce the heat to low, cover, and simmer for 25•30 minutes, or until the rice is tender and the liquid is absorbed.

To serve, divide the cooked brown rice and teriyaki chicken evenly among plates.

This teriyaki chicken with brown rice is a great option for a carb cycling diet plan. The brown rice provides a complex carbohydrate that is lower on the glycemic index, while the chicken is a lean protein source.

The teriyaki sauce adds flavor without significantly increasing the carb content. You can adjust the portion sizes of the rice and chicken to fit your specific carb cycling plan.

This dish is a balanced and satisfying meal that can be enjoyed as part of a carb cycling diet.

35. Egg fried rice with vegetables and chicken

Ingredient:

- 2 cups cooked brown rice, cooled
- 2 tbsp sesame oil, divided
- 2 eggs, beaten
- 1 lb boneless, skinless chicken breasts, diced
- 1 cup diced mixed vegetables (such as carrots, peas, and bell peppers)
- 2 cloves garlic, minced
- 1 tbsp low•sodium soy sauce
- 1 tsp rice vinegar
- Salt and pepper to taste
- Chopped green onions for garnish (optional)

Instructions:

1. Heat 1 tbsp of the sesame oil in a large skillet or wok over medium•high heat.

2. Add the beaten eggs and scramble them, breaking them up into small pieces as they cook. Remove the eggs from the skillet and set aside.

3. Add the remaining 1 tbsp of sesame oil to the skillet. Add the diced chicken and sauté for 5•7 minutes, until the chicken is cooked through.

4. Add the diced mixed vegetables and minced garlic to the skillet. Sauté for 3•4 minutes, until the vegetables are tender•crisp.

5. Add the cooked brown rice, soy sauce, and rice vinegar to the skillet. Stir to combine and heat through.

6. Gently fold the scrambled eggs back into the fried rice mixture.

7. Season the fried rice with salt and pepper to taste. Serve the egg fried rice hot, garnished with chopped green onions if desired.

This egg fried rice with vegetables and chicken is a great option for a carb cycling diet plan. The brown rice provides a complex carbohydrate, while the chicken and eggs offer protein. The vegetables add fiber and nutrients without significantly increasing the carb content.

You can adjust the portion sizes of the rice, chicken, and vegetables to fit your specific carb cycling plan. This dish is a flavorful and satisfying way to enjoy a healthier version of fried rice while following a carb cycling diet.

36. Chicken burrito bowl with rice, beans, and salsa

Ingredient:

- 1 lb boneless, skinless chicken breasts
- 1 tsp chili powder
- 1 tsp cumin
- 1 tsp garlic powder
- Salt and pepper to taste
- 1 cup cooked brown rice
- 1 (15 oz) can black beans, rinsed and drained
- 1 cup diced tomatoes or salsa
- 1/4 cup diced red onion
- 2 tbsp chopped fresh cilantro
- 1 avocado, diced (optional)
- Lime wedges for serving

Instructions:

1. Preheat your oven to 400°F (200°C).

2. Season the chicken breasts with the chili powder, cumin, garlic powder, salt, and pepper.

3. Place the seasoned chicken on a baking sheet and bake for 20•25 minutes, or until the chicken is cooked through and reaches an internal temperature of 165°F (74°C).

4. Once the chicken is cooked, shred or dice it.

5. In a bowl, layer the cooked brown rice, shredded chicken, black beans, diced tomatoes or salsa, red onion, and chopped cilantro.

6. Top with diced avocado, if desired. Serve the burrito bowl with lime wedges on the side.

This chicken burrito bowl is a great option for a carb cycling diet plan for a few reasons:

1. The brown rice provides a complex carbohydrate that is lower on the glycemic index.
2. The black beans add fiber and protein without too many net carbs.
3. The chicken, vegetables, and avocado (if used) provide healthy fats and nutrients.

You can adjust the portion sizes of the rice, chicken, beans, and toppings to fit your specific carb cycling plan. This dish is a flavorful and satisfying way to enjoy a Mexican•inspired meal while following a carb cycling diet.

37. Beef and broccoli over jasmine rice

Ingredient:

Beef and Broccoli:
- 1 lb flank steak, thinly sliced
- 2 tbsp low•sodium soy sauce
- 1 tbsp rice vinegar
- 1 tsp sesame oil
- 2 cloves garlic, minced
- 1 tbsp grated fresh ginger
- 2 cups broccoli florets
- 1 tbsp olive oil

Jasmine Rice:
- 1 cup uncooked jasmine rice
- 2 cups low•sodium chicken or vegetable broth

Instructions:

Beef and Broccoli:
1. In a large bowl, combine the sliced flank steak, soy sauce, rice vinegar, sesame oil, garlic, and ginger. Toss to coat the beef and let it marinate for 15•20 minutes.
2. Heat the olive oil in a large skillet or wok over high heat.
3. Add the marinated beef and stir•fry for 3•4 minutes, until the beef is browned and cooked through.
4. Add the broccoli florets to the skillet and continue to stir•fry for 2•3 minutes, until the broccoli is tender•crisp.

Jasmine Rice:
1. In a medium saucepan, combine the jasmine rice and chicken or vegetable broth.
2. Bring the mixture to a boil over high heat, then reduce the heat to low, cover, and simmer for 15•20 minutes, or until the rice is tender and the liquid is absorbed.

To serve, divide the cooked jasmine rice among plates and top with the beef and broccoli mixture.

This beef and broccoli with jasmine rice is a great option for a carb cycling diet plan. The jasmine rice provides a complex carbohydrate that is lower on the glycemic index, whlle the beef offers a lean protein source. The broccoli adds fiber and nutrients without significantly increasing the carb content.

You can adjust the portion sizes of the rice, beef, and broccoli to fit your specific carb cycling plan. This dish is a flavorful and satisfying way to enjoy a balanced meal while following a carb cycling diet.

38. Hawaiian poke bowl with rice and fresh fish

Ingredient:

- 1 cup cooked brown rice
- 8 oz sushi•grade tuna or salmon, diced
- 1/2 cup diced pineapple
- 1/2 cup diced cucumber
- 1/4 cup diced red onion
- 2 tbsp low•sodium soy sauce
- 1 tbsp sesame oil

- 1 tsp sesame seeds
- 1 tsp grated fresh ginger
- Salt and pepper to taste
- Sliced avocado (optional)
- Chopped green onions for garnish (optional)

Instructions:

1. In a medium bowl, combine the diced fish, pineapple, cucumber, and red onion.

2. In a small bowl, whisk together the soy sauce, sesame oil, sesame seeds, and grated ginger.

3. Pour the soy sauce mixture over the fish and vegetable mixture, and gently toss to coat.

4. Season the poke with salt and pepper to taste.

5. To assemble the bowls, divide the cooked brown rice among serving bowls.

6. Top the rice with the poke mixture.

7. If desired, add sliced avocado and chopped green onions as garnishes. Serve the Hawaiian poke bowls immediately.

This Hawaiian poke bowl is a great option for a carb cycling diet plan for a few reasons:

1. The brown rice provides a complex carbohydrate that is lower on the glycemic index.
2. The fresh fish, such as tuna or salmon, is a lean protein source.
3. The pineapple, cucumber, and avocado (if used) add fiber, vitamins, and healthy fats without significantly increasing the carb content.

You can adjust the portion sizes of the rice, fish, and vegetables to fit your specific carb cycling plan. This dish is a refreshing and nutritious way to enjoy a Hawaiian•inspired meal while following a carb cycling diet.

39. Turkey meatballs with quinoa

Ingredient:

- 1 lb ground turkey
- 1/2 cup cooked quinoa
- 1/4 cup diced onion
- 2 cloves garlic, minced
- 1 egg
- 2 tbsp parsley, chopped
- 1 tsp dried oregano
- 1/2 tsp salt
- 1/4 tsp black pepper

Instructions:

1. Preheat oven to 400°F. Line a baking sheet with parchment paper.

2. In a large bowl, combine the ground turkey, cooked quinoa, onion, garlic, egg, parsley, oregano, salt, and pepper. Mix well until fully incorporated.

3. Scoop the mixture by the tablespoon and roll into small meatballs, placing them on the prepared baking sheet.

4. Bake for 18•20 minutes, until the meatballs are cooked through and no longer pink in the center.

5. Serve the turkey meatballs over additional quinoa, roasted vegetables, or on their own.

This recipe is a great option for a carb cycling diet as it provides a lean protein source from the turkey, complex carbs from the quinoa, and minimal added fats. The meatballs can be enjoyed on higher carb days or lower carb days depending on your meal plan.

40. Stuffed acorn squash with wild rice and cranberries

Ingredient:

- 2 acorn squash, halved and seeded
- 1 cup cooked wild rice
- 1/2 cup dried cranberries
- 1/4 cup chopped pecans
- 2 tbsp chopped fresh parsley
- 1 tsp ground cinnamon
- 1/4 tsp ground nutmeg
- Salt and pepper to taste

Instructions:

1. Preheat oven to 400°F. Place the acorn squash halves cut•side up on a baking sheet. Bake for 30•40 minutes, until tender when pierced with a fork.

2. In a medium bowl, combine the cooked wild rice, dried cranberries, chopped pecans, parsley, cinnamon, and nutmeg. Season with salt and pepper.

3. Scoop the wild rice mixture evenly into the baked acorn squash halves.

4. Return the stuffed squash to the oven and bake for an additional 10•15 minutes, until heated through.

5. Serve the stuffed acorn squash warm.

This recipe is a great option for a carb cycling diet plan. The acorn squash provides complex carbs, while the wild rice, cranberries, and pecans add additional fiber and nutrients. It's a filling and satisfying dish that can be enjoyed on higher carb days. Adjust the portion size as needed to fit your daily carb intake goals.

41. Couscous salad with grilled vegetables

Ingredient:

- 1 cup dry couscous
- 1 cup boiling water
- 1 zucchini, sliced
- 1 red bell pepper, sliced
- 1 yellow squash, sliced
- 1 red onion, sliced
- 2 tbsp olive oil
- 1 tbsp balsamic vinegar
- 2 tbsp chopped fresh parsley
- 1 tbsp chopped fresh basil
- Salt and pepper to taste

Instructions:

1. Prepare the couscous according to package instructions. Fluff with a fork and set aside to cool.

2. Preheat grill or grill pan to medium•high heat. Toss the sliced zucchini, bell pepper, yellow squash, and red onion with 1 tbsp of the olive oil. Season with salt and pepper.

3. Grill the vegetables for 5•7 minutes per side, until tender and lightly charred. Remove from heat and let cool slightly.

4. In a large bowl, combine the cooked couscous, grilled vegetables, remaining 1 tbsp olive oil, balsamic vinegar, parsley, and basil. Toss to coat evenly.

5. Season the couscous salad with additional salt and pepper to taste.

6. Serve the couscous salad chilled or at room temperature.

This couscous salad is a great option for a carb cycling diet plan. The couscous provides complex carbs, while the grilled vegetables add fiber, vitamins, and minerals. Adjust the portion size as needed to fit your daily carb intake goals.

42. Chicken fajitas with whole wheat tortillas

Ingredient:

- 1 lb boneless, skinless chicken breasts, sliced into strips
- 1 red bell pepper, sliced
- 1 green bell pepper, sliced
- 1 onion, sliced
- 2 tbsp olive oil
- 2 tsp chili powder
- 1 tsp cumin
- 1 tsp garlic powder
- Salt and pepper to taste
- 8 whole wheat tortillas

Optional Toppings:
- Avocado
- Salsa
- Greek yogurt
- Shredded lettuce

Instructions:

1. In a large skillet or wok, heat the olive oil over medium•high heat.

2. Add the chicken strips, bell peppers, and onion. Season with chili powder, cumin, garlic powder, salt, and pepper.

3. Sauté the fajita mixture for 8•10 minutes, stirring occasionally, until the chicken is cooked through and the vegetables are tender.

4. Warm the whole wheat tortillas according to package instructions.

5. Serve the chicken fajita mixture in the warm tortillas. Top with desired toppings like avocado, salsa, Greek yogurt, and shredded lettuce.

This chicken fajita recipe is a great option for a carb cycling diet plan. The whole wheat tortillas provide complex carbs, while the chicken and vegetables offer lean protein and fiber. Adjust the portion sizes of the tortillas and toppings to fit your daily carb intake goals.

43. Mediterranean grilled lamb with couscous

Ingredient:

- 1 lb lamb loin chops or leg of lamb, cut into 1•inch cubes
- 2 tbsp olive oil
- 2 tsp dried oregano
- 1 tsp ground cumin
- 1 tsp paprika
- 1 garlic clove, minced
- Salt and pepper to taste
- 1 cup dry couscous
- 1 cup boiling water
- 1/2 cup diced cucumber
- 1/4 cup diced tomatoes
- 2 tbsp chopped fresh parsley
- 1 tbsp lemon juice
- 1 tbsp crumbled feta cheese (optional)

Instructions:

1. In a large bowl, combine the lamb cubes, olive oil, oregano, cumin, paprika, garlic, salt, and pepper. Toss to coat the lamb evenly. Cover and marinate for 30 minutes to 1 hour.

2. Preheat grill or grill pan to medium•high heat. Thread the marinated lamb onto skewers.

3. Grill the lamb skewers for 8•10 minutes, turning occasionally, until the lamb is cooked through and reaches your desired doneness.

4. While the lamb is grilling, prepare the couscous according to package instructions. Fluff with a fork and let cool slightly.

5. In a medium bowl, combine the cooked couscous, diced cucumber, tomatoes, parsley, and lemon juice. Toss to mix well.

6. Serve the grilled lamb skewers over the couscous salad. Top with crumbled feta cheese if desired.

This Mediterranean•inspired dish is a great option for a carb cycling diet plan. The couscous provides complex carbs, while the grilled lamb offers a lean protein source. Adjust the portion sizes to fit your daily carb intake goals.

44. Veggie-packed minestrone soup

Ingredient:

- 2 tbsp olive oil
- 1 onion, diced
- 3 carrots, diced
- 3 celery stalks, diced
- 3 garlic cloves, minced
- 1 tsp dried oregano
- 1 tsp dried basil
- 1/4 tsp red pepper flakes (optional)
- 1 (28 oz) can diced tomatoes
- 4 cups low-sodium vegetable or chicken broth
- 1 (15 oz) can kidney beans, rinsed and drained
- 1 (15 oz) can cannellini beans, rinsed and drained
- 2 cups chopped kale or spinach
- 1 cup small pasta (such as ditalini or elbow macaroni)
- Salt and pepper to taste
- Grated Parmesan cheese (optional)

Instructions:

1. In a large pot or Dutch oven, heat the olive oil over medium heat. Add the onion, carrots, celery, and garlic. Sauté for 5-7 minutes until the vegetables are softened.

2. Stir in the oregano, basil, and red pepper flakes (if using). Cook for 1 minute until fragrant.

3. Add the diced tomatoes, vegetable or chicken broth, kidney beans, and cannellini beans. Bring the soup to a simmer.

4. Stir in the chopped kale or spinach and the small pasta. Simmer for 10-15 minutes, or until the pasta is tender.

5. Season the soup with salt and pepper to taste.

6. Serve the minestrone soup hot, topped with grated Parmesan cheese if desired.

This veggie-packed minestrone soup is a great option for a carb cycling diet plan. It's loaded with fiber-rich vegetables, beans for protein, and a small amount of pasta for complex carbs. Adjust the portion size as needed to fit your daily carb intake goals.

45. Whole wheat wrap with grilled chicken and veggies

Ingredient:

- 4 oz boneless, skinless chicken breasts
- 1 tbsp olive oil
- 1 tsp dried Italian seasoning
- Salt and pepper to taste
- 1 whole wheat tortilla or wrap
- 1/2 cup mixed grilled vegetables (such as zucchini, bell peppers, onions)
- 2 tbsp hummus
- 1/4 cup baby spinach or arugula

Instructions:

1. Preheat grill or grill pan to medium•high heat.

2. Brush the chicken breasts with 1 tsp of the olive oil and season with the Italian seasoning, salt, and pepper.

3. Grill the chicken for 5•7 minutes per side, until cooked through. Remove from heat and let rest for a few minutes, then slice or shred the chicken.

4. In a separate grill basket or on skewers, grill the mixed vegetables with the remaining 1 tsp of olive oil until tender and lightly charred, about 8•10 minutes.

5. Warm the whole wheat tortilla or wrap according to package instructions.

6. Spread the hummus evenly over the center of the wrap. Top with the grilled chicken, grilled vegetables, and baby spinach or arugula.

7. Fold the bottom of the wrap up, then fold in the sides and roll up tightly to create a wrap.

8. Serve immediately.

This whole wheat wrap with grilled chicken and veggies is a great option for a carb cycling diet plan. The whole wheat wrap provides complex carbs, while the chicken and vegetables offer lean protein and fiber. Adjust the portion size as needed to fit your daily carb intake goals.

46. Barley risotto with mushrooms and Parmesan

Ingredient:

- 1 cup pearl barley
- 4 cups low•sodium vegetable or chicken broth
- 1 tbsp olive oil
- 8 oz sliced mushrooms
- 1 onion, diced
- 2 garlic cloves, minced
- 1/2 cup dry white wine (optional)
- 1/2 cup grated Parmesan cheese
- 2 tbsp chopped fresh parsley
- Salt and pepper to taste

Instructions:

1. In a medium saucepan, bring the vegetable or chicken broth to a simmer. Add the pearl barley, cover, and cook for 25•30 minutes, until the barley is tender. Drain any excess liquid and set aside.

2. In a large skillet, heat the olive oil over medium heat. Add the sliced mushrooms and sauté for 5•7 minutes, until they start to brown.

3. Add the diced onion and minced garlic to the skillet. Cook for 2•3 minutes, until the onion is translucent.

4. Pour in the white wine (if using) and let it simmer for 1•2 minutes to deglaze the pan.

5. Add the cooked barley to the skillet with the mushrooms and onions. Stir to combine.

6. Stir in the grated Parmesan cheese and chopped parsley. Season with salt and pepper to taste.

7. Serve the barley risotto warm.

This barley risotto dish is a great option for a carb cycling diet plan. Barley is a whole grain that provides complex carbs, while the mushrooms and Parmesan add flavor and nutrients without too many additional carbs. Adjust the portion size as needed to fit your daily carb intake goals.

47. Chicken and vegetable kebabs with quinoa

Ingredient:

- 1 lb boneless, skinless chicken breasts, cut into 1•inch cubes
- 1 red bell pepper, cut into 1•inch pieces
- 1 zucchini, cut into 1•inch pieces
- 1 red onion, cut into 1•inch pieces
- 2 tbsp olive oil
- 1 tsp dried oregano
- 1 tsp garlic powder
- Salt and pepper to taste
- 1 cup dry quinoa, cooked according to package instructions

For the Marinade:
- 2 tbsp olive oil
- 2 tbsp lemon juice
- 1 tbsp Dijon mustard
- 1 garlic clove, minced
- 1 tsp dried oregano
- Salt and pepper to taste

Instructions:

1. In a shallow dish, whisk together the marinade ingredients. Add the chicken cubes and toss to coat. Cover and refrigerate for 30 minutes to 1 hour.

2. Preheat grill or grill pan to medium•high heat.

3. Thread the marinated chicken, bell pepper, zucchini, and onion onto skewers.

4. In a small bowl, combine the 2 tbsp olive oil, oregano, garlic powder, salt, and pepper. Brush this mixture over the kebabs.

5. Grill the kebabs for 12•15 minutes, turning occasionally, until the chicken is cooked through and the vegetables are tender.

6. Serve the grilled chicken and vegetable kebabs over the cooked quinoa.

This chicken and vegetable kebab dish is a great option for a carb cycling diet plan. The quinoa provides complex carbs, while the lean chicken and grilled vegetables offer protein and fiber. Adjust the portion sizes to fit your daily carb intake goals.

48. Tuna pasta salad with whole wheat pasta

Ingredient:

- 8 oz whole wheat pasta (such as penne or fusilli)
- 2 (5 oz) cans tuna, drained
- 1 cup diced cucumber
- 1 cup cherry tomatoes, halved
- 1/2 cup diced red onion
- 1/4 cup chopped fresh parsley
- 2 tbsp olive oil
- 2 tbsp lemon juice
- 1 tsp Dijon mustard
- Salt and pepper to taste

Instructions:

1. Cook the whole wheat pasta according to package instructions. Drain and rinse with cold water to cool.

2. In a large bowl, combine the cooked and cooled pasta, tuna, cucumber, cherry tomatoes, red onion, and parsley.

3. In a small bowl, whisk together the olive oil, lemon juice, and Dijon mustard. Season with salt and pepper.

4. Pour the dressing over the pasta salad and toss gently to coat everything evenly.

5. Refrigerate the tuna pasta salad for at least 30 minutes to allow the flavors to meld.

6. Serve chilled or at room temperature.

This tuna pasta salad is a great option for a carb cycling diet plan. The whole wheat pasta provides complex carbs, while the tuna adds lean protein. The vegetables and lemon•Dijon dressing add flavor and nutrients without too many additional carbs. Adjust the portion size as needed to fit your daily carb intake goals.

49. *Asian-style noodle soup with tofu and vegetables*

Ingredient:

- 4 cups low-sodium vegetable or chicken broth
- 2 tbsp low-sodium soy sauce
- 1 tbsp rice vinegar
- 1 tsp sesame oil
- 1 tsp grated fresh ginger
- 1 garlic clove, minced
- 8 oz firm or extra-firm tofu, cubed
- 2 cups mixed vegetables (such as sliced mushrooms, snow peas, shredded cabbage, carrots)
- 4 oz whole wheat or brown rice noodles
- 2 green onions, sliced
- Chopped cilantro for garnish (optional)

Instructions:

1. In a large saucepan, combine the vegetable or chicken broth, soy sauce, rice vinegar, sesame oil, grated ginger, and minced garlic. Bring to a simmer over medium heat.

2. Add the cubed tofu and mixed vegetables to the simmering broth. Cook for 5-7 minutes, until the vegetables are tender.

3. Add the whole wheat or brown rice noodles to the soup and cook for an additional 3-5 minutes, until the noodles are tender.

4. Remove from heat and stir in the sliced green onions.

5. Ladle the noodle soup into bowls and garnish with chopped cilantro, if desired.

This Asian-style noodle soup is a great option for a carb cycling diet plan. The whole wheat or brown rice noodles provide complex carbs, while the tofu and vegetables offer protein and fiber. Adjust the portion size as needed to fit your daily carb intake goals.

50. Pork stir-fry with soba noodles

Ingredient:

- 8 oz soba noodles
- 1 lb pork tenderloin, thinly sliced
- 2 tbsp low•sodium soy sauce
- 1 tbsp rice vinegar
- 1 tsp sesame oil
- 1 tbsp grated fresh ginger
- 2 garlic cloves, minced
- 2 tbsp olive oil
- 2 cups mixed stir•fry vegetables (such as broccoli, bell peppers, snow peas, carrots)
- 2 green onions, sliced
- Sesame seeds for garnish (optional)

Sauce:
- 2 tbsp low•sodium soy sauce
- 1 tbsp rice vinegar
- 1 tsp honey
- 1 tsp cornstarch

Instructions:

1. Cook the soba noodles according to package instructions. Drain and rinse with cold water.

2. In a small bowl, combine the 2 tbsp soy sauce, 1 tbsp rice vinegar, 1 tsp sesame oil, grated ginger, and minced garlic. Add the pork slices and toss to coat. Let marinate for 15•20 minutes.

3. In another small bowl, whisk together the sauce ingredients (2 tbsp soy sauce, 1 tbsp rice vinegar, honey, and cornstarch).

4. Heat the olive oil in a large skillet or wok over high heat. Add the marinated pork and stir•fry for 3•4 minutes until lightly browned.

5. Add the mixed stir•fry vegetables to the skillet and continue to stir•fry for 3•4 minutes, until the vegetables are tender•crisp.

6. Pour the sauce into the skillet and bring to a simmer, stirring constantly, until the sauce thickens, about 1•2 minutes.

7. Add the cooked soba noodles and toss everything together until well combined. Serve the pork and vegetable stir•fry with soba noodles, garnished with sliced green onions and sesame seeds if desired.

This pork stir•fry with soba noodles is a great option for a carb cycling diet plan. The soba noodles provide complex carbs, while the pork and vegetables offer protein and fiber. Adjust the portion sizes to fit your daily carb intake goals.

51. Spaghetti carbonara

Ingredient:

- 8 oz whole wheat spaghetti
- 4 slices center•cut bacon, diced
- 2 eggs
- 1/2 cup grated Parmesan cheese
- 1/4 cup low•fat milk
- 2 garlic cloves, minced
- 1/4 tsp black pepper
- 2 tbsp chopped fresh parsley

Instructions:

1. Bring a large pot of salted water to a boil. Cook the whole wheat spaghetti according to package instructions until al dente. Drain and set aside.

2. In a large skillet, cook the diced bacon over medium heat until crispy, about 5•7 minutes. Remove the bacon from the pan and set aside, reserving the bacon fat in the skillet.

3. In a medium bowl, whisk together the eggs, Parmesan cheese, milk, garlic, and black pepper.

4. Add the cooked spaghetti to the skillet with the bacon fat. Toss the pasta to coat it in the fat.

5. Remove the skillet from the heat and quickly pour the egg mixture over the hot pasta, tossing constantly to coat the noodles. The residual heat from the pasta will cook the eggs and create a creamy sauce.

6. Stir in the cooked bacon and chopped parsley.

7. Serve the spaghetti carbonara immediately, while hot.

This spaghetti carbonara recipe is a great option for a carb cycling diet plan. The whole wheat spaghetti provides complex carbs, while the eggs, Parmesan, and bacon add protein. Adjust the portion size as needed to fit your daily carb intake goals.

52. Baked potato with sour cream and chives

Ingredient:

- 4 medium russet potatoes
- 1/4 cup low•fat sour cream
- 2 tbsp chopped fresh chives
- Salt and pepper to taste

Instructions:

1. Preheat the oven to 400°F.

2. Scrub the potatoes and prick them several times with a fork. Place the potatoes directly on the oven rack and bake for 50•60 minutes, until tender when pierced with a fork.

3. Remove the potatoes from the oven and let them cool for 5 minutes.

4. Cut each potato in half lengthwise. Scoop out the flesh into a bowl, leaving a thin layer of potato attached to the skin.

5. Mash the potato flesh with a fork or potato masher. Stir in the low•fat sour cream and chopped chives. Season with salt and pepper to taste.

6. Spoon the mashed potato mixture back into the potato skins.

7. Serve the stuffed baked potatoes warm.

This baked potato dish is a great option for a carb cycling diet plan. The potato provides complex carbs, while the sour cream and chives add flavor without too many additional carbs. Adjust the portion size as needed to fit your daily carb intake goals.

53. Beef lasagna

Ingredient:

- 8 oz whole wheat lasagna noodles
- 1 lb lean ground beef
- 1 onion, diced
- 3 garlic cloves, minced
- 1 (28 oz) can crushed tomatoes
- 2 tbsp tomato paste
- 1 tsp dried oregano
- 1/2 tsp dried basil
- Salt and pepper to taste
- 1 cup low•fat ricotta cheese
- 1 egg
- 1/2 cup grated Parmesan cheese
- 2 cups shredded part•skim mozzarella cheese

Instructions:

1. Preheat the oven to 375°F.

2. Bring a large pot of salted water to a boil. Cook the whole wheat lasagna noodles according to package instructions until al dente. Drain and set aside.

3. In a large skillet, cook the ground beef over medium heat until browned and crumbled, about 5•7 minutes. Drain any excess fat.

4. Add the diced onion and minced garlic to the skillet. Sauté for 2•3 minutes until the onion is translucent.

5. Stir in the crushed tomatoes, tomato paste, oregano, and basil. Season with salt and pepper. Simmer the sauce for 10•15 minutes.

6. In a medium bowl, mix together the ricotta cheese, egg, and 1/4 cup of the Parmesan cheese.

7. Spread 1 cup of the meat sauce in the bottom of a 9x13 inch baking dish. Layer 3•4 lasagna noodles over the sauce. Spread half of the ricotta cheese mixture over the noodles, then top with 1 cup of the meat sauce and 1/2 cup of the mozzarella cheese.

8. Repeat the layers of noodles, ricotta, meat sauce, and mozzarella cheese. Top with the remaining lasagna noodles and the remaining meat sauce. Sprinkle the top with the remaining Parmesan cheese.

9. Cover the dish with foil and bake for 30 minutes. Remove the foil and bake for an additional 15•20 minutes, until the cheese is melted and bubbly. Let the lasagna cool for 10•15 minutes before serving.

This beef lasagna recipe can be a great option for a carb cycling diet plan. The whole wheat noodles provide complex carbs, while the lean ground beef and low•fat cheeses offer protein. Adjust the portion size as needed to fit your daily carb intake goals.

54. Chicken and rice casserole

Ingredient:

- 1 cup uncooked brown rice
- 1 lb boneless, skinless chicken breasts, cubed
- 1 onion, diced
- 2 cups sliced mushrooms
- 1 cup frozen peas
- 1 (10.5 oz) can low•sodium cream of mushroom soup
- 1/2 cup low•fat milk
- 1/4 cup grated Parmesan cheese
- 1 tsp dried thyme
- Salt and pepper to taste

Instructions:

1. Preheat the oven to 375°F.

2. Cook the brown rice according to package instructions. Set aside.

3. In a large skillet, sauté the diced onion over medium heat until translucent, about 5 minutes.

4. Add the cubed chicken to the skillet and cook until no longer pink, about 7•10 minutes.

5. Stir in the sliced mushrooms and frozen peas. Cook for an additional 3•5 minutes.

6. In a medium bowl, whisk together the cream of mushroom soup and low•fat milk.

7. In a 9x13 inch baking dish, layer the cooked brown rice, chicken and vegetable mixture, and the soup mixture. Sprinkle the top with the grated Parmesan cheese and dried thyme.

8. Bake the casserole for 25•30 minutes, until the cheese is melted and the edges are bubbly. Let the casserole cool for 5•10 minutes before serving.

This chicken and rice casserole is a great option for a carb cycling diet plan. The brown rice provides complex carbs, while the chicken, vegetables, and low•fat dairy ingredients offer protein and nutrients. Adjust the portion size as needed to fit your daily carb intake goals.

55. Vegetable pizza with thin crust

Ingredient:

- 1 cup whole wheat flour
- 1 tsp active dry yeast
- 1/2 tsp salt
- 1/2 cup warm water
- 1 tbsp olive oil
- 1 cup marinara or pizza sauce
- 1 cup mixed vegetables (such as sliced bell peppers, mushrooms, onions, spinach)
- 1 cup shredded part•skim mozzarella cheese

Instructions:

1. In a medium bowl, combine the whole wheat flour, yeast, and salt. Add the warm water and olive oil, and stir until a dough forms.

2. Turn the dough out onto a lightly floured surface and knead for 2•3 minutes until smooth and elastic.

3. Roll or stretch the dough into a thin, 12•inch circle on a baking sheet or pizza pan.

4. Preheat the oven to 400°F.

5. Spread the marinara or pizza sauce evenly over the dough, leaving a 1/2•inch border.

6. Top the pizza with the mixed vegetables, distributing them evenly.

7. Sprinkle the shredded mozzarella cheese over the top.

8. Bake the pizza for 15•18 minutes, until the crust is golden brown and the cheese is melted and bubbly. Let the pizza cool for 5 minutes before slicing and serving.

This vegetable pizza with a thin whole wheat crust is a great option for a carb cycling diet plan. The whole wheat crust provides complex carbs, while the vegetables and cheese offer protein and nutrients. Adjust the portion size as needed to fit your daily carb intake goals.

56. Pad Thai with shrimp

Ingredient:

- 8 oz rice noodles
- 2 tbsp low•sodium soy sauce
- 2 tbsp rice vinegar
- 1 tbsp honey
- 1 tsp sesame oil
- 1 lb peeled and deveined shrimp
- 2 tbsp olive oil
- 2 garlic cloves, minced
- 1 cup shredded cabbage
- 1 cup bean sprouts
- 2 green onions, sliced
- 2 tbsp chopped roasted peanuts (optional)
- Lime wedges for serving

Instructions:

1. Soak the rice noodles in hot water for 15•20 minutes, until softened. Drain and set aside.

2. In a small bowl, whisk together the soy sauce, rice vinegar, honey, and sesame oil. Set aside.

3. In a large skillet or wok, heat the olive oil over medium•high heat. Add the shrimp and garlic, and sauté for 2•3 minutes until the shrimp are partially cooked.

4. Add the softened rice noodles and the soy sauce mixture to the skillet. Toss everything together and cook for 2•3 minutes, until the noodles are tender and the shrimp are cooked through.

5. Stir in the shredded cabbage, bean sprouts, and green onions. Cook for an additional 1•2 minutes, until the vegetables are slightly wilted.

6. Remove the Pad Thai from heat and serve immediately, garnished with chopped roasted peanuts (if using) and lime wedges.

This Pad Thai with shrimp is a great option for a carb cycling diet plan. The rice noodles provide complex carbs, while the shrimp and vegetables offer protein and fiber. Adjust the portion size as needed to fit your daily carb intake goals.

57. Vegetable Biryani

Ingredient:

- 1 cup basmati rice
- 2 tbsp olive oil
- 1 onion, diced
- 3 garlic cloves, minced
- 1 tbsp grated fresh ginger
- 1 tsp garam masala
- 1 tsp ground cumin
- 1 tsp ground coriander
- 1/2 tsp turmeric
- 1/4 tsp cayenne pepper (optional)

- 1 cup mixed vegetables (such as cauliflower, bell peppers, peas, carrots)
- 1 (15 oz) can chickpeas, rinsed and drained
- 1 cup low•sodium vegetable broth
- 1/4 cup chopped fresh cilantro
- Salt and pepper to taste
- Lemon wedges for serving

Instructions:

1. Cook the basmati rice according to package instructions. Fluff with a fork and set aside.

2. In a large skillet or Dutch oven, heat the olive oil over medium heat. Add the diced onion and sauté for 5•7 minutes until translucent.

3. Stir in the minced garlic and grated ginger. Cook for 1•2 minutes until fragrant.

4. Add the garam masala, cumin, coriander, turmeric, and cayenne (if using). Stir to coat the onions and cook for 1 minute.

5. Add the mixed vegetables and chickpeas to the skillet. Pour in the vegetable broth and stir to combine.

6. Bring the mixture to a simmer, then reduce heat to low, cover, and cook for 15•20 minutes, until the vegetables are tender.

7. Stir the cooked basmati rice into the vegetable mixture. Taste and adjust seasoning with salt and pepper as needed. Remove from heat and stir in the chopped fresh cilantro. Serve the vegetable biryani warm, with lemon wedges on the side.

This vegetable biryani is a great option for a carb cycling diet plan. The basmati rice provides complex carbs, while the vegetables and chickpeas offer fiber and protein. Adjust the portion size as needed to fit your daily carb intake goals.

58. Cheeseburger with bun and sweet potato fries

Ingredient:

- 1 lb lean ground beef
- 4 whole wheat hamburger buns
- 4 slices low•fat cheddar cheese
- Lettuce, tomato, onion, pickles (optional toppings)
- 2 medium sweet potatoes, cut into 1/2•inch thick fries
- 1 tbsp olive oil
- 1 tsp paprika
- Salt and pepper to taste

Instructions:

1. Preheat oven to 400°F.

2. Form the ground beef into 4 equal•sized patties, about 4•5 inches wide and 1/2•inch thick. Season with salt and pepper.

3. Heat a grill or grill pan over medium•high heat. Cook the burgers for 3•4 minutes per side, until cooked through. During the last minute of cooking, top each burger with a slice of low•fat cheddar cheese.

4. Toast the whole wheat hamburger buns.

5. On a large baking sheet, toss the sweet potato fries with the olive oil, paprika, salt, and pepper.

6. Bake the sweet potato fries for 20•25 minutes, flipping halfway, until crispy.

7. Assemble the cheeseburgers by placing the patty on the bottom bun, then adding your desired toppings.

8. Serve the cheeseburgers with the baked sweet potato fries on the side.

This cheeseburger and sweet potato fries meal is a great option for a carb cycling diet plan. The whole wheat bun provides complex carbs, while the lean beef, cheese, and sweet potato fries offer a balance of protein, carbs, and healthy fats. Adjust the portion sizes as needed to fit your daily carb intake goals.

59. Pancakes with maple syrup and berries

Ingredient:

- 1 cup whole wheat flour
- 1 tsp baking powder
- 1/4 tsp baking soda
- 1/4 tsp salt
- 1 egg
- 1 cup low•fat milk
- 1 tbsp honey
- 1 tsp vanilla extract
- 1 cup fresh or frozen berries (such as blueberries, raspberries, or strawberries)
- 2 tbsp pure maple syrup

Instructions:

1. In a medium bowl, whisk together the whole wheat flour, baking powder, baking soda, and salt.

2. In a separate bowl, whisk the egg, milk, honey, and vanilla extract.

3. Pour the wet ingredients into the dry ingredients and stir just until combined (do not overmix).

4. Heat a nonstick skillet or griddle over medium heat. Lightly grease the surface.

5. For each pancake, pour about 1/4 cup of the batter onto the hot surface. Sprinkle a few berries on top.

6. Cook the pancakes for 2•3 minutes per side, until golden brown.

7. Serve the whole wheat pancakes warm, drizzled with 1•2 teaspoons of pure maple syrup per serving.

This whole wheat pancake recipe is a great option for a carb cycling diet plan. The whole wheat flour provides complex carbs, while the berries and maple syrup add natural sweetness without too many additional carbs. Adjust the portion size as needed to fit your daily carb intake goals.

60. Chicken quesadillas with flour tortillas

Ingredient:

- 8 oz boneless, skinless chicken breasts, grilled and shredded
- 4 (8•inch) whole wheat flour tortillas
- 1 cup shredded low•fat cheddar or Monterey Jack cheese
- 1/2 cup diced bell peppers
- 1/4 cup diced onion
- 1 tbsp olive oil
- Salt and pepper to taste
- Salsa, guacamole, or low•fat sour cream for serving (optional)

Instructions:

1. In a skillet over medium heat, sauté the diced bell peppers and onion in the olive oil for 3•4 minutes until softened.

2. Add the shredded chicken to the skillet and season with salt and pepper. Stir to combine and heat through.

3. Place one tortilla in a large skillet or griddle over medium heat. Sprinkle 1/4 cup of the shredded cheese evenly over half of the tortilla.

4. Top the cheese with 1/4 of the chicken and vegetable mixture.

5. Fold the other half of the tortilla over the filling to create a half•moon shape.

6. Cook the quesadilla for 2•3 minutes per side, until the tortilla is lightly browned and the cheese is melted.

7. Repeat the process with the remaining 3 tortillas, cheese, and chicken•vegetable filling.

8. Cut each quesadilla in half and serve warm, with salsa, guacamole, or low•fat sour cream on the side if desired.

This chicken quesadilla recipe is a great option for a carb cycling diet plan. The whole wheat flour tortillas provide complex carbs, while the chicken, cheese, and vegetables offer protein and fiber. Adjust the portion size as needed to fit your daily carb intake goals.

61. Beef tacos with corn tortillas

Ingredient:

- 1 lb lean ground beef
- 1 tbsp chili powder
- 1 tsp ground cumin
- 1/2 tsp garlic powder
- 1/2 tsp onion powder
- 1/4 tsp cayenne pepper (optional)
- Salt and pepper to taste
- 12 small corn tortillas
- 1 cup shredded lettuce
- 1/2 cup diced tomatoes
- 1/4 cup diced onion
- 1/4 cup shredded low•fat cheddar cheese
- Lime wedges for serving

Instructions:

1. In a large skillet over medium•high heat, cook the ground beef, breaking it up with a wooden spoon, until browned and cooked through, about 5•7 minutes.

2. Drain any excess fat from the skillet. Stir in the chili powder, cumin, garlic powder, onion powder, and cayenne (if using). Season with salt and pepper.

3. Warm the corn tortillas according to package instructions, either in a dry skillet or wrapped in a damp paper towel and microwaved for 20•30 seconds.

4. To assemble the tacos, place a couple of tablespoons of the seasoned ground beef in the center of each warm corn tortilla.

5. Top the beef with shredded lettuce, diced tomatoes, diced onion, and a sprinkle of shredded low•fat cheddar cheese.

6. Serve the beef tacos immediately, with lime wedges on the side.

This beef taco recipe is a great option for a carb cycling diet plan. The corn tortillas provide complex carbs, while the lean ground beef, lettuce, tomatoes, and cheese offer protein, fiber, and nutrients. Adjust the portion size as needed to fit your daily carb intake goals.

62. Pita bread with falafel and tahini sauce

Ingredient:

For the Tahini Sauce:
• 1/4 cup tahini
• 2 tbsp lemon juice
• 1 garlic clove, minced
• 2•3 tbsp water
• Salt and pepper to taste

For Serving:
• 4 whole wheat pita breads, halved
• 1 cup chopped tomatoes
• 1/2 cup chopped cucumber
• 1/4 cup chopped red onion

For the Falafel:
• 1 (15 oz) can chickpeas, rinsed and drained
• 1/2 cup chopped parsley
• 2 garlic cloves, minced
• 1 tsp ground cumin
• 1/2 tsp ground coriander
• 1/4 tsp cayenne pepper
• 2 tbsp whole wheat flour
• 1 tbsp olive oil

Instructions:

1. Make the falafel: In a food processor, combine the chickpeas, parsley, garlic, cumin, coriander, and cayenne. Pulse until a coarse paste forms. Transfer to a bowl and stir in the whole wheat flour.

2. Form the chickpea mixture into small balls, about 1•2 tablespoons each. Heat the olive oil in a skillet over medium heat. Fry the falafel for 2•3 minutes per side until golden brown.

3. Make the tahini sauce: In a small bowl, whisk together the tahini, lemon juice, garlic, and 2•3 tablespoons of water until a smooth, pourable sauce forms. Season with salt and pepper.

4. To assemble, place the falafel inside the pita bread halves. Top with chopped tomatoes, cucumber, and red onion. Drizzle the tahini sauce over the top.

5. Serve the pita bread with falafel and tahini sauce immediately.

This pita bread with falafel and tahini sauce is a great option for a carb cycling diet plan. The whole wheat pita provides complex carbs, while the falafel and tahini sauce offer protein and healthy fats. Adjust the portion size as needed to fit your daily carb intake goals.

63. Macaroni and cheese

Ingredient:

- 8 oz whole wheat elbow macaroni
- 2 tbsp olive oil
- 2 tbsp whole wheat flour
- 2 cups low•fat milk
- 1 cup shredded low•fat cheddar cheese
- 1/4 cup grated Parmesan cheese
- 1/4 tsp ground mustard
- 1/4 tsp paprika
- Salt and pepper to taste
- 1/4 cup whole wheat breadcrumbs (optional)

Instructions:

1. Bring a large pot of salted water to a boil. Cook the whole wheat elbow macaroni according to package instructions until al dente. Drain and set aside.

2. In a medium saucepan, heat the olive oil over medium heat. Whisk in the whole wheat flour and cook for 1•2 minutes, stirring constantly.

3. Gradually whisk in the low•fat milk. Bring the mixture to a simmer and cook, stirring frequently, until thickened, about 5•7 minutes.

4. Remove the saucepan from heat and stir in the shredded low•fat cheddar cheese, Parmesan cheese, ground mustard, and paprika. Season with salt and pepper to taste.

5. Add the cooked whole wheat macaroni to the cheese sauce and stir to combine.

6. Transfer the macaroni and cheese to a baking dish. If desired, top with the whole wheat breadcrumbs.

7. Bake at 375°F for 15•20 minutes, until the breadcrumbs are golden brown and the cheese is bubbly.

8. Let the macaroni and cheese cool for 5 minutes before serving.

This carb•friendly macaroni and cheese is a great option for a carb cycling diet plan. The whole wheat pasta provides complex carbs, while the reduced•fat cheese and milk keep the dish relatively low in additional carbs. Adjust the portion size as needed to fit your daily carb intake goals.

64. Chicken Alfredo pasta

Ingredient:

- 8 oz whole wheat fettuccine pasta
- 1 lb boneless, skinless chicken breasts, grilled and sliced
- 2 tbsp olive oil
- 2 garlic cloves, minced
- 2 tbsp whole wheat flour
- 1 cup low•fat milk
- 1/2 cup grated Parmesan cheese
- 1/4 cup low•fat plain Greek yogurt
- 1/4 tsp ground nutmeg
- Salt and pepper to taste
- 2 cups steamed broccoli florets (optional)

Instructions:

1. Bring a large pot of salted water to a boil. Cook the whole wheat fettuccine according to package instructions until al dente. Drain and set aside.

2. In a large skillet, heat the olive oil over medium heat. Add the minced garlic and cook for 1 minute until fragrant.

3. Sprinkle the whole wheat flour over the garlic and whisk to create a roux. Cook for 1•2 minutes, stirring constantly.

4. Gradually whisk in the low•fat milk and bring the mixture to a simmer. Cook, stirring frequently, until the sauce thickens, about 5•7 minutes.

5. Remove the skillet from heat and stir in the grated Parmesan cheese, Greek yogurt, and ground nutmeg. Season with salt and pepper to taste.

6. Add the cooked whole wheat fettuccine and sliced grilled chicken to the Alfredo sauce. Toss to coat everything evenly.

7. If desired, stir in the steamed broccoli florets. Serve the chicken Alfredo pasta warm.

This chicken Alfredo pasta recipe is a great option for a carb cycling diet plan. The whole wheat fettuccine provides complex carbs, while the chicken, Parmesan, and Greek yogurt offer protein and healthy fats. Adjust the portion size as needed to fit your daily carb intake goals.

65. Naan bread with butter chicken

Ingredient:

For the Butter Chicken:
- 1 lb boneless, skinless chicken thighs, cubed
- 2 tbsp olive oil
- 1 onion, diced
- 3 garlic cloves, minced
- 1 tbsp grated fresh ginger
- 1 tsp garam masala
- 1 tsp ground cumin
- 1 tsp paprika
- 1/2 tsp cayenne pepper (optional)
- 1 (15 oz) can diced tomatoes
- 1/2 cup low•fat plain Greek yogurt
- 2 tbsp tomato paste
- 1/4 cup heavy cream or coconut milk
- Salt and pepper to taste

For the Naan Bread:
- 1 cup whole wheat flour
- 1/2 cup low•fat plain Greek yogurt
- 1 tsp baking powder
- 1/4 tsp salt
- 1 tbsp melted butter or ghee (optional)

Instructions:

1. Make the butter chicken: In a large skillet, heat the olive oil over medium•high heat. Add the cubed chicken and sauté until browned on all sides, about 5•7 minutes. Remove the chicken from the skillet and set aside.

2. In the same skillet, sauté the diced onion for 3•4 minutes until translucent. Add the minced garlic and grated ginger, and cook for 1 minute more.

3. Stir in the garam masala, cumin, paprika, and cayenne (if using). Cook for 1 minute to toast the spices.

4. Pour in the diced tomatoes, Greek yogurt, and tomato paste. Bring the mixture to a simmer and cook for 5•7 minutes, until slightly thickened.

5. Return the sautéed chicken to the skillet and stir in the heavy cream or coconut milk. Simmer for 10•15 minutes, until the chicken is cooked through. Season with salt and pepper to taste.

6. Make the naan bread: In a medium bowl, whisk together the whole wheat flour, Greek yogurt, baking powder, and salt until a shaggy dough forms.

7. Turn the dough out onto a lightly floured surface and knead for 2•3 minutes until smooth and elastic. Divide the dough into 4 equal pieces. Use a rolling pin to roll each piece into a thin, oval•shaped naan.

9. Heat a large skillet or griddle over medium•high heat. Cook the naan for 2•3 minutes per side, until lightly charred and puffed. Brush the warm naan with melted butter or ghee, if desired. Serve the butter chicken warm, with the freshly baked naan bread.

66. Cheese and spinach stuffed manicotti

Ingredient:

- 8 oz whole wheat manicotti pasta shells
- 1 cup part•skim ricotta cheese
- 1 cup shredded part•skim mozzarella cheese
- 1/4 cup grated Parmesan cheese
- 1 egg
- 2 cups fresh spinach, chopped
- 1 garlic clove, minced
- 1/4 tsp dried oregano
- 1/4 tsp dried basil
- Salt and pepper to taste
- 1 (24 oz) jar low•sugar marinara sauce

Instructions:

1. Preheat the oven to 375°F.

2. Cook the whole wheat manicotti shells according to package instructions until al dente. Drain and set aside.

3. In a medium bowl, mix together the ricotta cheese, 1/2 cup of the mozzarella cheese, Parmesan cheese, egg, chopped spinach, minced garlic, oregano, and basil. Season with salt and pepper.

4. Stuff the ricotta•spinach mixture into the cooked manicotti shells, using a spoon or piping bag.

5. Spread 1 cup of the marinara sauce in the bottom of a 9x13 inch baking dish.

6. Arrange the stuffed manicotti shells in a single layer in the baking dish. Pour the remaining marinara sauce over the top.

7. Sprinkle the remaining 1/2 cup of mozzarella cheese over the top.

8. Bake for 25•30 minutes, until the cheese is melted and bubbly. Let the stuffed manicotti cool for 5 minutes before serving.

This cheese and spinach stuffed manicotti is a great option for a carb cycling diet plan. The whole wheat pasta provides complex carbs, while the ricotta, mozzarella, and spinach offer protein and nutrients. Adjust the portion size as needed to fit your daily carb intake goals.

67. Gnocchi with tomato sauce

Ingredient:

- 1 lb russet potatoes, peeled and cut into 1•inch cubes
- 1 egg, lightly beaten
- 1/2 cup all•purpose flour, plus more for dusting
- 1/4 tsp salt
- 1 tbsp olive oil
- 1 (28 oz) can crushed tomatoes
- 2 cloves garlic, minced
- 1 tsp dried oregano
- 1/4 tsp red pepper flakes (optional)
- Salt and pepper to taste
- Grated Parmesan cheese for serving (optional)

Instructions:

1. Place the potato cubes in a pot and cover with water. Bring to a boil and cook until tender, about 15 minutes. Drain and mash the potatoes until smooth.

2. Allow the potatoes to cool slightly, then mix in the egg, 1/2 cup flour, and 1/4 tsp salt until a soft dough forms.

3. Lightly flour a clean surface and gently roll the dough into long 1/2•inch thick ropes. Cut the ropes into 1•inch pieces to form the gnocchi.

4. Bring a large pot of salted water to a boil. Working in batches, gently drop the gnocchi into the boiling water and cook until they float to the top, about 2•3 minutes. Remove with a slotted spoon.

5. In a skillet, heat the olive oil over medium heat. Add the garlic and cook for 1 minute until fragrant.

6. Add the crushed tomatoes, oregano, and red pepper flakes (if using). Season with salt and pepper. Simmer for 5•10 minutes.

7. Add the cooked gnocchi to the tomato sauce and gently toss to coat. Serve immediately, topped with grated Parmesan cheese if desired.

This gnocchi dish is a great carb•focused meal that can be enjoyed as part of a carb cycling diet plan. Adjust portion sizes as needed to fit your macros.

68. Vegetable tempura with dipping sauce

Ingredient:

For the Tempura:
- 1 cup all•purpose flour
- 1 tbsp cornstarch
- 1 tsp baking powder
- 1/2 tsp salt
- 1 cup cold seltzer water or club soda
- Assorted vegetables (such as sliced zucchini, sweet potato, bell pepper, broccoli florets)
- Vegetable oil for frying

For the Dipping Sauce:
- 1/4 cup low•sodium soy sauce
- 2 tbsp rice vinegar
- 1 tbsp honey
- 1 tsp sesame oil
- 1 tsp grated ginger
- 1 clove garlic, minced
- 1/4 tsp red pepper flakes (optional)

Instructions:

1. Make the dipping sauce by combining all the sauce ingredients in a small bowl. Set aside.

2. In a medium bowl, whisk together the flour, cornstarch, baking powder and salt. Slowly whisk in the cold seltzer water until a light, airy batter forms. Do not overmix.

3. Heat 2•3 inches of vegetable oil in a large pot or Dutch oven to 350°F.

4. Working in batches, dip the vegetable pieces into the tempura batter, allowing any excess to drip off. Carefully lower the battered veggies into the hot oil and fry for 2•3 minutes until golden brown and crispy.

5. Remove the tempura with a slotted spoon and drain on a paper towel•lined plate. Season lightly with salt. Serve the hot tempura immediately with the dipping sauce on the side. Enjoy!

This tempura makes a great carb•focused side dish or appetizer. The light, crispy batter and fresh vegetables pair perfectly with the flavorful dipping sauce. Adjust portion sizes as needed to fit your carb cycling macros.

69. Risotto with butternut squash and sage

Ingredient:

- 1 lb butternut squash, peeled, seeded and cut into 1/2•inch cubes
- 2 tbsp olive oil, divided
- 1 onion, finely chopped
- 2 cloves garlic, minced
- 1 cup Arborio rice
- 1/2 cup dry white wine
- 4 cups low•sodium chicken or vegetable broth, heated
- 2 tbsp chopped fresh sage, plus more for garnish
- 2 tbsp grated Parmesan cheese
- Salt and pepper to taste

Instructions:

1. Preheat oven to 400°F. Toss the cubed butternut squash with 1 tbsp olive oil on a baking sheet. Roast for 20•25 minutes, until tender and lightly browned. Set aside.

2. In a large skillet or Dutch oven, heat the remaining 1 tbsp olive oil over medium heat. Add the onion and cook for 5 minutes until translucent.

3. Add the garlic and Arborio rice. Cook for 2•3 minutes, stirring frequently, until the rice is lightly toasted.

4. Pour in the white wine and cook, stirring constantly, until the wine is absorbed, about 2 minutes.

5. Add the hot broth 1/2 cup at a time, stirring constantly, until the liquid is absorbed before adding more. Continue this process until the rice is tender and creamy, about 20•25 minutes total.

6. Stir in the roasted butternut squash, chopped sage, and Parmesan. Season with salt and pepper to taste. Serve the risotto immediately, garnished with additional fresh sage leaves if desired.

This risotto makes a hearty, carb•focused main dish. The butternut squash and sage add wonderful fall flavors. Adjust portion sizes as needed to fit your carb cycling macros.

70. Sweet and sour chicken with white rice

Ingredient:

For the Chicken:
• 1 lb boneless, skinless chicken breasts, cut into 1•inch pieces
• 2 tbsp cornstarch
• 2 tbsp olive oil

For the Sauce:
• 1/4 cup low•sodium soy sauce
• 2 tbsp rice vinegar
• 2 tbsp honey
• 1 tbsp tomato paste
• 1 tsp sesame oil
• 1/4 tsp red pepper flakes (optional)

For the Vegetables:
• 1 red bell pepper, cut into 1•inch pieces
• 1 cup pineapple chunks (fresh or canned, drained)
• 2 green onions, sliced

For the Rice:
• 1 cup uncooked white rice
• 2 cups low•sodium chicken broth

Instructions:

1. Cook the rice: In a medium saucepan, bring the chicken broth to a boil. Add the rice, cover and reduce heat to low. Simmer for 15•20 minutes until rice is tender. Fluff with a fork.

2. Make the sauce: In a small bowl, whisk together the soy sauce, vinegar, honey, tomato paste, sesame oil and red pepper flakes (if using). Set aside.

3. Prepare the chicken: In a medium bowl, toss the chicken pieces with the cornstarch until evenly coated.

4. Heat the olive oil in a large skillet or wok over medium•high heat. Add the chicken and cook for 5•7 minutes, stirring occasionally, until browned and cooked through.

5. Add the bell pepper, pineapple and sauce to the skillet. Bring to a simmer and cook for 2•3 minutes, until the sauce thickens slightly.

6. Remove from heat and stir in the sliced green onions. Serve the sweet and sour chicken immediately over the cooked white rice.

This sweet and sour chicken dish makes a great carb•focused meal. Adjust portion sizes as needed to fit your carb cycling macros.

71. Cornbread with chili con carne

Ingredient:

For the Chili:
- 1 lb ground beef or ground turkey
- 1 onion, diced
- 3 cloves garlic, minced
- 2 tbsp chili powder
- 1 tsp ground cumin
- 1 tsp dried oregano
- 1/2 tsp smoked paprika
- 1/4 tsp cayenne pepper (optional)
- 1 (15 oz) can diced tomatoes
- 1 (15 oz) can kidney beans, drained and rinsed
- 1 cup low•sodium beef or chicken broth
- Salt and pepper to taste

For the Cornbread:
- 1 cup cornmeal
- 1 cup all•purpose flour
- 2 tsp baking powder
- 1/2 tsp salt
- 1 egg
- 1 cup low•fat milk
- 2 tbsp honey
- 2 tbsp unsalted butter, melted

Instructions:

1. Make the chili: In a large pot or Dutch oven, cook the ground beef/turkey over medium•high heat until browned and crumbled, 5•7 minutes. Drain excess fat.

2. Add the onion and garlic to the pot and cook for 2•3 minutes until softened.

3. Stir in the chili powder, cumin, oregano, paprika, and cayenne (if using). Cook for 1 minute.

4. Pour in the diced tomatoes, kidney beans, and broth. Season with salt and pepper. Bring to a simmer and let cook for 15•20 minutes, until thickened.

5. Make the cornbread: Preheat oven to 400°F. Grease an 8•inch square baking pan.

6. In a medium bowl, whisk together the cornmeal, flour, baking powder and salt.

7. In a separate bowl, beat the egg. Then whisk in the milk, honey and melted butter. Pour the wet ingredients into the dry ingredients and stir just until combined (do not overmix).

8. Spread the cornbread batter into the prepared pan. Bake for 18•22 minutes, until golden brown and a toothpick inserted in the center comes out clean. Serve the chili con carne warm, with slices of the cornbread on the side.

72. Chicken pot pie with puff pastry

Ingredient:

For the Filling:
• 1 lb boneless, skinless chicken breasts,
cut into 1•inch pieces
• 2 tbsp olive oil
• 1 onion, diced
• 2 carrots, peeled and diced
• 2 celery stalks, diced
• 8 oz cremini mushrooms, sliced
• 2 garlic cloves, minced

• 2 tbsp all•purpose flour
• 1 cup low•sodium chicken broth
• 1/2 cup unsweetened almond milk
• 1 tsp dried thyme
• 1/2 tsp dried rosemary
• Salt and pepper to taste

For the Topping:
• 1 sheet frozen puff pastry, thawed

Instructions:

1. Preheat oven to 400°F.

2. In a large skillet, heat the olive oil over medium•high heat. Add the chicken and cook for 5•7 minutes until browned on all sides. Remove chicken from skillet and set aside.

3. Add the onion, carrots, celery and mushrooms to the skillet. Cook for 5•7 minutes until vegetables are tender.

4. Stir in the garlic and cook for 1 minute until fragrant.

5. Sprinkle the flour over the vegetables and stir to coat. Cook for 2 minutes.

6. Gradually whisk in the chicken broth and almond milk. Bring to a simmer and cook for 5 minutes, until thickened.

7. Return the cooked chicken to the skillet. Stir in the thyme, rosemary, salt and pepper.

8. Transfer the chicken filling to a 9•inch pie dish or baking dish.

9. Unfold the puff pastry sheet and place it over the filling, pressing the edges to seal. Cut a few slits in the top to allow steam to escape.

10. Bake for 25•30 minutes, until the puff pastry is golden brown. Let cool for 5 minutes before serving

73. Jambalaya with sausage and shrimp

Ingredient:

- 1 lb andouille sausage, sliced into 1/2•inch pieces
- 1 lb peeled and deveined shrimp
- 1 tbsp olive oil
- 1 onion, diced
- 1 bell pepper, diced
- 2 celery stalks, diced
- 3 garlic cloves, minced
- 1 (14.5 oz) can diced tomatoes
- 1 cup low•sodium chicken broth
- 1 cup uncooked long•grain white rice
- 1 tsp smoked paprika
- 1 tsp dried oregano
- 1/2 tsp cayenne pepper (optional)
- Salt and pepper to taste
- Chopped parsley for garnish

Instructions:

1. In a large skillet or Dutch oven, cook the sausage over medium•high heat for 5•7 minutes until browned. Remove sausage from pan and set aside.

2. Add the olive oil to the pan. Sauté the onion, bell pepper, celery and garlic for 5 minutes until softened.

3. Stir in the diced tomatoes, chicken broth, rice, smoked paprika, oregano and cayenne (if using). Season with salt and pepper.

4. Bring the mixture to a boil, then reduce heat to low, cover and simmer for 15•20 minutes, until the rice is tender.

5. Stir the cooked sausage and shrimp into the jambalaya. Cover and cook for 5•7 minutes more, until the shrimp are opaque and cooked through.

6. Remove from heat and let stand for 5 minutes. Fluff the jambalaya with a fork and serve immediately, garnished with chopped parsley.

This jambalaya makes a hearty, carb•focused one•dish meal. The sausage and shrimp provide protein, while the rice and vegetables make it a balanced dish. Adjust portion sizes as needed to fit your carb cycling macros.

74. Fettuccine primavera

Ingredient:

- 8 oz whole wheat fettuccine pasta
- 1 tbsp olive oil
- 1 cup broccoli florets
- 1 cup sliced zucchini
- 1 cup sliced mushrooms
- 1 red bell pepper, sliced
- 3 cloves garlic, minced
- 1/2 cup low•sodium chicken or vegetable broth
- 2 tbsp grated Parmesan cheese
- 2 tbsp chopped fresh parsley
- Salt and pepper to taste

Instructions:

1. Bring a large pot of salted water to a boil. Cook the fettuccine according to package instructions until al dente. Drain and set aside.

2. In a large skillet, heat the olive oil over medium•high heat. Add the broccoli, zucchini, mushrooms and bell pepper. Sauté for 5•7 minutes until vegetables are tender•crisp.

3. Add the garlic to the skillet and cook for 1 minute until fragrant.

4. Pour in the broth and bring to a simmer. Cook for 2•3 minutes to allow the flavors to meld.

5. Add the cooked fettuccine to the skillet and toss everything together until the pasta is well coated.

6. Remove from heat and stir in the Parmesan cheese and chopped parsley.

7. Season with salt and pepper to taste. Serve the fettuccine primavera immediately.

This primavera dish makes a great carb•focused meal. The whole wheat fettuccine and variety of fresh vegetables provide fiber and nutrients. Adjust portion sizes as needed to fit your carb cycling macros.

75. Stuffed crepes with ricotta and berries

Ingredient:

For the Crepes:
- 3 eggs
- 1 cup unsweetened almond milk
- 1/2 cup whole wheat flour
- 1 tbsp honey
- 1/4 tsp salt

For the Filling:
- 1 cup part•skim ricotta cheese
- 1/4 cup fresh berries (such as raspberries, blueberries or blackberries)
- 1 tbsp honey
- 1/2 tsp vanilla extract

Instructions:

1. Make the crepes: In a blender, combine the eggs, almond milk, flour, honey and salt. Blend until smooth.

2. Heat a small non•stick skillet or crepe pan over medium heat. Lightly grease the pan with non•stick cooking spray.

3. Pour about 2•3 tbsp of the crepe batter into the pan, tilting and swirling to evenly coat the bottom. Cook for 1•2 minutes until the edges start to lightly brown.

4. Carefully flip the crepe and cook for another 30 seconds to 1 minute. Transfer to a plate and repeat with remaining batter to make 8•10 crepes total.

5. Make the filling: In a small bowl, mix together the ricotta, berries, honey and vanilla until well combined.

6. To assemble, place a crepe on a flat surface. Spoon about 2•3 tbsp of the ricotta filling into the center. Fold the sides of the crepe over the filling and roll up.

7. Place the stuffed crepe seam•side down on a serving plate. Repeat with remaining crepes and filling. Serve the stuffed crepes immediately, or refrigerate until ready to serve.

This crepe dish makes a delicious carb•focused breakfast or dessert. The ricotta and berries provide protein and nutrients to balance out the carbs from the crepes. Adjust portion sizes as needed to fit your carb cycling macros.

76. Greek yogurt with honey and almonds

Ingredient:
- 1 cup plain Greek yogurt
- 1 tbsp honey
- 2 tbsp sliced almonds

Instructions:

1. Scoop the Greek yogurt into a serving bowl.

2. Drizzle the honey over the top of the yogurt.

3. Sprinkle the sliced almonds over the honey.

4. Serve immediately.

That's it! This simple yogurt parfait is a great carb•conscious snack or light breakfast option.

The Greek yogurt provides protein, while the honey adds a touch of sweetness. The almonds contribute healthy fats and a nice crunch.

This can be easily adjusted to fit your carb cycling macros. You can use more or less yogurt, honey, and almonds depending on your needs.

Some variations to try:

- Top with fresh berries
- Swap the honey for a small amount of maple syrup or agave
- Use different nuts like walnuts or pecans
- Add a sprinkle of cinnamon or vanilla extract

The key is to keep the portions controlled and the ingredients simple and nutrient•dense. This makes for a satisfying, carb•friendly snack or breakfast.

77. Cottage cheese with pineapple

Ingredient:
- 1 cup low•fat or non•fat cottage cheese
- 1/2 cup fresh pineapple chunks
- 1 tsp honey (optional)

Instructions:

1. Scoop the cottage cheese into a small bowl.

2. Top the cottage cheese with the fresh pineapple chunks.

3. If desired, drizzle the honey over the top.

That's it! This simple cottage cheese and pineapple dish makes a great carb•conscious snack or light meal.

The cottage cheese provides a good amount of protein, while the pineapple adds natural sweetness and a dose of vitamin C. The honey is optional, but can add a touch more sweetness if desired.

This is a very flexible recipe • you can adjust the amounts of cottage cheese and pineapple to suit your macros and preferences. Some other variations to try:

- Use canned pineapple tidbits instead of fresh
- Top with a sprinkle of cinnamon or nutmeg
- Add a handful of chopped nuts like almonds or walnuts
- Swap the pineapple for other fresh fruit like berries or diced mango

The key is to keep the portions controlled and the ingredients simple and nutrient•dense. This makes for a satisfying, carb•friendly snack that can be enjoyed as part of a carb cycling diet plan.

78. Mixed nuts

Ingredient:

- 1/4 cup raw almonds
- 1/4 cup raw walnuts
- 1/4 cup raw cashews
- 1/4 cup raw pecans
- 1/4 tsp sea salt (optional)

Instructions:

1. In a small bowl, combine the almonds, walnuts, cashews, and pecans.

2. If desired, sprinkle the mixed nuts with a light dusting of sea salt and toss to coat.

3. Serve the mixed nuts immediately or store in an airtight container at room temperature for up to 1 week.

This simple mixed nuts snack is a great option for a carb cycling diet plan. Nuts are high in healthy fats and protein, making them a filling and nutritious snack.

The combination of different nuts provides a variety of nutrients, flavors, and textures. You can adjust the ratios of each nut to your preference.

The salt is optional, but a light sprinkle can help enhance the natural flavors of the nuts.

Be mindful of portion sizes, as nuts are calorie•dense. A 1/4 cup serving is a good guideline for this mixed nuts snack. Adjust the serving size as needed to fit your carb cycling macros.

This makes a great portable, shelf•stable snack to have on hand. Pair it with some fresh fruit or a small amount of plain Greek yogurt for a more substantial carb•conscious treat.

79. Hummus with carrot sticks

Ingredient:

For the Hummus:
- 1 (15 oz) can chickpeas, drained and rinsed
- 2 tbsp tahini
- 2 tbsp fresh lemon juice
- 1 garlic clove, minced
- 2 tbsp olive oil
- 2•3 tbsp water
- 1/4 tsp ground cumin
- 1/4 tsp paprika
- Salt and pepper to taste

For the Carrot Sticks: 4•5 medium carrots, peeled and cut into sticks

Instructions:

1. Make the hummus: In a food processor, combine the chickpeas, tahini, lemon juice, garlic, olive oil, 2 tbsp water, cumin and paprika. Blend until smooth, adding more water as needed to reach desired consistency.

2. Season the hummus with salt and pepper to taste.

3. Transfer the hummus to a serving bowl.

4. Prepare the carrot sticks by peeling and cutting the carrots into long, thin sticks.

5. Serve the hummus immediately with the carrot sticks for dipping.

This homemade hummus and carrot sticks make a great carb•conscious snack. The chickpeas in the hummus provide protein and fiber, while the carrots are a low•carb, nutrient•dense vegetable.

You can adjust the portion sizes of the hummus and carrot sticks to fit your carb cycling macros. Some other veggie options to serve with the hummus include celery sticks, cucumber slices, or bell pepper strips.

This is a simple, healthy snack that can be easily prepared ahead of time. Store any leftover hummus in an airtight container in the refrigerator for up to 5 days.

80. Avocado toast on whole grain bread

Ingredient:

- 2 slices whole grain or sprouted bread
- 1 ripe avocado, mashed
- 1 tbsp olive oil
- 1 tsp lemon juice
- 1/4 tsp salt
- 1/8 tsp black pepper
- Red pepper flakes (optional)

Instructions:

1. Toast the two slices of whole grain bread until lightly golden brown.

2. In a small bowl, mash the avocado with a fork. Stir in the olive oil, lemon juice, salt and black pepper until well combined.

3. Spread the mashed avocado mixture evenly over the toasted bread slices.

4. If desired, sprinkle a pinch of red pepper flakes over the top of the avocado toast.

5. Serve immediately.

This avocado toast makes a great carb•focused breakfast or snack. The whole grain bread provides complex carbs, while the avocado adds healthy fats and fiber to help keep you feeling full.

You can adjust the portion sizes to fit your carb cycling macros. For example, you could have one slice of toast as a snack or two slices as part of a larger meal.

Some variations to try:

- Top with a fried or poached egg
- Sprinkle with chopped tomatoes, onions or fresh herbs
- Drizzle with a bit of balsamic glaze
- Use a different type of whole grain bread like rye or sourdough

The key is to choose high•quality, nutrient•dense ingredients that will provide sustained energy and keep you satisfied as part of your carb cycling diet plan.

81. Apple slices with peanut butter

Ingredient:

- 1 medium apple, cored and sliced
- 2 tbsp natural peanut butter (no added sugar)

Instructions:

1. Wash and slice the apple into thin wedges or slices.

2. Spread 1•2 teaspoons of peanut butter onto each apple slice.

That's it! This simple snack is a great option for a carb cycling diet.

The apple provides complex carbs, fiber, and natural sweetness, while the peanut butter adds protein and healthy fats to help keep you feeling full and satisfied.

You can adjust the portion sizes to fit your individual carb cycling macros. For example, you could have 4•5 apple slices with 1•2 tbsp of peanut butter as a snack.

Some variations to try:

- Use a different type of nut butter, such as almond or cashew butter
- Sprinkle a pinch of cinnamon over the top
- Drizzle a small amount of honey over the peanut butter
- Pair with a small handful of raw nuts or seeds

The key is to choose high•quality, minimally processed ingredients that will provide a balance of macronutrients to support your carb cycling goals.

This apple and peanut butter snack is portable, easy to prepare, and can be enjoyed anytime as part of a healthy carb cycling diet plan.

82. Protein smoothie with berries and spinach

Ingredient:

- 1 cup unsweetened almond milk
- 1/2 cup frozen mixed berries (such as blueberries, raspberries, blackberries)
- 1 scoop vanilla protein powder
- 1 cup fresh spinach leaves
- 1 tbsp almond butter
- 1 tsp honey (optional)
- Ice cubes (as needed)

Instructions:

1. Add the almond milk, frozen berries, protein powder, spinach, almond butter, and honey (if using) to a high•powered blender.

2. Blend on high speed until the mixture is smooth and creamy, about 1•2 minutes. Add ice cubes as needed to reach desired consistency.

3. Pour the smoothie into a glass and enjoy immediately.

This protein•packed smoothie is a great option for a carb cycling diet plan. The combination of berries, spinach, and protein powder provides a nutrient•dense, low•carb treat.

The almond milk and almond butter add healthy fats to help keep you feeling full, while the honey (if used) provides a touch of natural sweetness.

You can adjust the amounts of each ingredient to fit your specific carb cycling macros. For example, you could use less almond milk for a thicker consistency, or add more or less protein powder depending on your needs.

Some other variations to try:

- Swap the berries for other low•carb fruits like raspberries or blackberries
- Use Greek yogurt instead of almond milk for extra protein
- Add a handful of kale or other greens instead of spinach
- Top with a sprinkle of cinnamon or unsweetened coconut flakes

This smoothie makes a great carb•conscious breakfast, snack, or post•workout recovery drink. Enjoy it as part of your balanced carb cycling diet plan.

83. Hard-boiled eggs

Ingredient:

• 6 large eggs

Instructions:

1. Place the eggs in a single layer in a saucepan and cover with cold water by 1 inch.

2. Bring the water to a boil over high heat. Once the water reaches a full boil, remove the pan from the heat and cover.

3. Let the eggs sit in the hot water for the following times:
• For soft•boiled eggs: 6•7 minutes
• For hard•boiled eggs: 12 minutes

4. Drain the hot water and cover the eggs with cold water to stop the cooking. Let sit for 5 minutes.

5. Peel the eggs and enjoy immediately or refrigerate in an airtight container for up to 1 week.

Hard•boiled eggs are a fantastic protein•rich snack that fits perfectly into a carb cycling diet plan. They are easy to prepare in advance and provide a convenient, portable option.

Each large hard•boiled egg contains about 6 grams of protein and less than 1 gram of carbs, making them an ideal low•carb food choice.

You can enjoy hard•boiled eggs on their own as a snack, or incorporate them into other dishes like salads, avocado toast, or veggie wraps.

Some tips for perfect hard•boiled eggs:

• Use eggs that are a few days old, as they are easier to peel
• Add a teaspoon of baking soda to the cooking water to help with peeling
• Shock the cooked eggs in an ice bath to make peeling even easier

Hard•boiled eggs are a versatile, nutrient•dense food that can be a great addition to your carb cycling meal plan. Adjust portion sizes as needed to fit your macros.

84. Edamame

Ingredient:

- 1 lb frozen edamame in the pod
- 1 tsp coarse sea salt (optional)

Instructions:

1. Bring a large pot of salted water to a boil over high heat.

2. Add the frozen edamame pods to the boiling water. Cook for 5•7 minutes, until the pods are bright green and tender.

3. Drain the edamame and transfer to a serving bowl.

4. If desired, sprinkle the cooked edamame with the coarse sea salt.

5. Serve the edamame warm, providing small bowls for guests to shell and eat the beans.

Edamame is a great carb•conscious snack or side dish that fits well into a carb cycling diet plan. The soybeans provide a good amount of plant•based protein, fiber, and nutrients.

Each 1/2 cup serving of shelled edamame contains around 9 grams of carbs, making it a relatively low•carb option. The salt is optional, but can help enhance the natural flavors.

Some tips for enjoying edamame:

- Look for pre•shelled edamame to save time and effort
- Experiment with different seasonings like garlic powder, lemon pepper, or chili lime seasoning
- Serve edamame as a snack with veggie sticks or whole grain crackers
- Add cooked edamame to salads, rice dishes, or stir•fries

Edamame is a versatile, nutrient•dense food that can be a great addition to your carb cycling meal plan. Adjust portion sizes as needed to fit your macros.

85. Cheese and crackers

Ingredient:

- 1 oz (about 2•3 slices) low•fat cheddar or mozzarella cheese
- 6•8 whole grain crackers

Instructions:

1. Slice or cube the cheese into bite•sized pieces.

2. Arrange the cheese pieces and crackers on a small plate or in a snack•sized container.

This cheese and crackers snack is a great option for a carb cycling diet plan. It provides a balance of protein, complex carbs, and healthy fats to help keep you feeling satisfied.

The key is to choose high•quality, minimally processed ingredients:

- Opt for low•fat or reduced•fat cheese to keep the calories and fat in check.
- Select whole grain crackers that are higher in fiber and lower in added sugars.
- Avoid processed cheese products and highly refined crackers.

A typical serving size would be 1 oz of cheese (about 2•3 thin slices) paired with 6•8 whole grain crackers. This provides around 12•15 grams of carbs, depending on the specific crackers used.

You can easily adjust the portion sizes to fit your individual carb cycling macros. For example, you could have a smaller serving as a snack or a larger serving as part of a meal.

Some variations to try:

- Use different types of cheese like cheddar, mozzarella, or goat cheese
- Add a small amount of nuts or seeds for extra healthy fats
- Pair the cheese and crackers with fresh fruit or veggie sticks
- Spread a thin layer of hummus or nut butter on the crackers

This simple cheese and crackers snack is portable, satisfying, and can be a great addition to your carb cycling diet plan.

86. Trail mix with dried fruit and nuts

Ingredient:

- 1/4 cup raw almonds
- 1/4 cup raw walnuts
- 2 tbsp unsweetened coconut flakes
- 2 tbsp pumpkin seeds
- 2 tbsp dried cranberries
- 2 tbsp unsweetened dried cherries

Instructions:

1. In a medium bowl, combine all the ingredients and mix well.

2. Transfer the trail mix to an airtight container or resealable bag.

This trail mix makes a great portable, carb•conscious snack option for a carb cycling diet plan. The combination of nuts, seeds, and dried fruit provides a balance of healthy fats, protein, and complex carbs.

Here's a breakdown of the nutritional profile:

- Nuts and seeds provide healthy fats and protein to help keep you feeling full.
- Dried fruit adds natural sweetness and carbs, but in moderation.
- Unsweetened coconut flakes contribute fiber and healthy fats.

A typical serving size is 1/4 cup, which contains around 15•20 grams of carbs, depending on the specific ingredients used.

You can easily adjust the ratios of nuts, seeds, and dried fruit to suit your individual carb cycling macros. Some variations to try:

- Use different nuts like pecans, cashews or pistachios
- Swap the dried cranberries and cherries for other low•sugar dried fruits like blueberries or apricots
- Add a sprinkle of cinnamon or a pinch of sea salt
- Include a small amount of dark chocolate chips or cacao nibs

This homemade trail mix is a great way to satisfy your snack cravings while staying on track with your carb cycling plan. Store it in an airtight container for up to 2 weeks.

87. Dark chocolate (moderation)

Ingredient:

- 4 oz high•quality dark chocolate (70•85% cacao)
- 1 tbsp coconut oil
- 1 tsp vanilla extract
- Pinch of sea salt

Instructions:

1. Line a small baking dish or plate with parchment paper.

2. In a double boiler or heatproof bowl set over a pot of simmering water, melt the dark chocolate and coconut oil, stirring frequently until smooth.

3. Remove from heat and stir in the vanilla extract and sea salt.

4. Pour the chocolate mixture into the prepared baking dish and spread evenly.

5. Refrigerate for 30 minutes to 1 hour, until set.

6. Once set, remove from the refrigerator and cut into small squares, about 1•inch each.

7. Store the dark chocolate squares in an airtight container in the refrigerator for up to 2 weeks.

Enjoy 1•2 squares of this rich, dark chocolate as a treat in moderation. The coconut oil and vanilla add a nice flavor complexity. Be mindful of portion sizes, as dark chocolate is high in calories and fat, though the antioxidants can provide some health benefits in small amounts.

88. Rice cakes with almond butter

Ingredient:

- 2 whole grain brown rice cakes
- 2 tbsp all•natural almond butter
- 1 tsp honey (optional)

Instructions:

1. Spread 1 tbsp of almond butter evenly over each rice cake.

2. Drizzle 1/2 tsp of honey over the almond butter on each rice cake, if desired. The honey adds a touch of sweetness.

3. Enjoy the rice cakes as a snack or light meal. The combination of the complex carbs from the rice cakes and the healthy fats and protein from the almond butter makes this a great option for a carb cycling diet.

Nutrition Info (per serving):
- Calories: 200
- Carbs: 18g
- Protein: 7g
- Fat: 12g
- Fiber: 3g

This snack is perfect for a lower carb day on a carb cycling plan. The rice cakes provide a satisfying crunch while the almond butter adds healthy fats and protein to keep you feeling full. Adjust the portion size as needed to fit your individual macros for the day.

89. Fruit salad with yogurt

Ingredient:

- 1 cup mixed fresh fruit (such as strawberries, blueberries, pineapple, mango)
- 1/2 cup plain Greek yogurt
- 1 tsp honey (optional)
- 1 tbsp chopped nuts (such as almonds or walnuts)

Instructions:

1. In a medium bowl, gently toss together the mixed fruit.

2. Top the fruit with the plain Greek yogurt. Drizzle with honey if desired to add a touch of sweetness.

3. Sprinkle the chopped nuts over the top.

4. Serve chilled or at room temperature.

Nutrition Info (per serving):
- Calories: 150
- Carbs: 20g
- Protein: 10g
- Fat: 5g
- Fiber: 3g

This fruit salad with yogurt makes a great option for a higher carb day on a carb cycling plan. The natural sugars from the fruit provide carbs, while the Greek yogurt adds protein and probiotics. The nuts add a crunchy texture and healthy fats. Adjust the portion sizes as needed to fit your individual macros.

90. Baked apple with cinnamon

Ingredient:

- 2 medium apples, cored and halved
- 1 tsp ground cinnamon
- 1 tbsp honey (optional)
- 2 tbsp water

Instructions:

1. Preheat the oven to 375°F.

2. Place the apple halves in a baking dish. Sprinkle the cinnamon evenly over the top of the apples.

3. Drizzle the honey over the apples, if using. The honey adds a touch of sweetness.

4. Pour the water into the bottom of the baking dish.

5. Bake for 20•25 minutes, until the apples are tender when pierced with a fork.

6. Serve the baked apples warm.

Nutrition Info (per serving):
- Calories: 80
- Carbs: 20g
- Protein: 0g
- Fat: 0g
- Fiber: 3g

This baked apple dish makes a great option for a higher carb day on a carb cycling plan. The natural sweetness from the apples provides carbs, while the cinnamon adds flavor without extra calories or sugar. Adjust the portion size as needed to fit your individual macros for the day.

91. Chia pudding with coconut milk

Ingredient:

- 1/4 cup chia seeds
- 1 cup unsweetened coconut milk
- 1 tsp vanilla extract
- 1 tbsp honey (optional)
- Fresh berries for topping (optional)

Instructions:

1. In a medium bowl, whisk together the chia seeds, coconut milk, and vanilla extract until well combined.

2. Cover the bowl and refrigerate for at least 2 hours, or overnight, stirring occasionally, until the mixture has thickened to a pudding•like consistency.

3. If using, stir in the honey to sweeten the pudding.

4. Serve the chia pudding chilled, topped with fresh berries if desired.

Nutrition Info (per serving):
- Calories: 200
- Carbs: 15g
- Protein: 5g
- Fat: 15g
- Fiber: 8g

This chia pudding makes a great option for a lower carb day on a carb cycling plan. The chia seeds provide fiber, protein, and healthy fats, while the coconut milk adds creaminess. Adjust the portion size as needed to fit your individual macros for the day.

92. Frozen yogurt with fresh fruit

Ingredient:

- 1 cup plain Greek yogurt
- 1 tbsp honey (optional)
- 1 cup mixed fresh fruit (such as berries, mango, pineapple)

Instructions:

1. In a medium bowl, stir together the Greek yogurt and honey (if using) until well combined.

2. Pour the yogurt mixture into an ice cube tray or small ramekins. Freeze for 2•3 hours, until firm.

3. Once frozen, pop the yogurt cubes out of the tray or ramekins.

4. Arrange the frozen yogurt cubes in a bowl and top with the fresh mixed fruit.

Nutrition Info (per serving):
- Calories: 150
- Carbs: 20g
- Protein: 10g
- Fat: 2g
- Fiber: 3g

This frozen yogurt with fresh fruit makes a great option for a higher carb day on a carb cycling plan. The natural sugars from the fruit provide carbs, while the Greek yogurt adds protein and probiotics. Adjust the portion sizes as needed to fit your individual macros for the day.

93. Popcorn (lightly salted)

Ingredient:

- 1/4 cup unpopped popcorn kernels
- 1 tsp olive oil or avocado oil
- 1/4 tsp sea salt

Instructions:

1. In a large pot with a tight•fitting lid, heat the oil over medium•high heat.

2. Add the popcorn kernels in an even layer. Cover the pot and wait for the popping to begin.

3. Once the popping starts, shake the pot gently to prevent burning. Continue popping until the popping slows to 2•3 seconds between pops.

4. Remove the pot from the heat and transfer the popped popcorn to a large bowl.

5. Sprinkle the sea salt over the popcorn and toss to coat evenly.

Nutrition Info (per serving, 3 cups popped):
- Calories: 100
- Carbs: 15g
- Protein: 3g
- Fat: 3g
- Fiber: 3g

This lightly salted popcorn makes a great option for a higher carb day on a carb cycling plan. The complex carbs from the popcorn provide sustained energy, while the minimal added salt keeps it a healthy snack. Adjust the portion size as needed to fit your individual macros for the day.

94. Whole grain toast with avocado

Ingredient:

- 2 slices whole grain bread
- 1/2 ripe avocado, mashed
- 1 tsp olive oil
- 1/4 tsp sea salt
- 1/4 tsp ground black pepper

Instructions:

1. Toast the whole grain bread until lightly golden brown.

2. In a small bowl, mash the avocado with the olive oil, sea salt, and black pepper until well combined.

3. Spread the mashed avocado evenly over the toasted whole grain bread slices.

4. Serve immediately.

Nutrition Info (per serving):
- Calories: 200
- Carbs: 20g
- Protein: 6g
- Fat: 12g
- Fiber: 6g

This whole grain toast with avocado makes a great option for a lower carb day on a carb cycling plan. The whole grain bread provides complex carbs, while the avocado adds healthy fats and fiber to keep you feeling full. Adjust the portion size as needed to fit your individual macros for the day.

95. Berry parfait with granola

Ingredient:

- 1 cup mixed berries (such as blueberries, raspberries, strawberries)
- 1 cup plain Greek yogurt
- 1/4 cup low•sugar granola

Instructions:

1. In a parfait glass or small bowl, layer half of the mixed berries on the bottom.

2. Top the berries with half of the Greek yogurt.

3. Sprinkle half of the granola over the yogurt.

4. Repeat the layers, ending with the granola on top.

Nutrition Info (per serving):
- Calories: 200
- Carbs: 25g
- Protein: 15g
- Fat: 5g
- Fiber: 5g

This berry parfait with granola makes a great option for a higher carb day on a carb cycling plan. The natural sugars from the berries provide carbs, while the Greek yogurt adds protein and the granola adds a crunchy texture. Adjust the portion size as needed to fit your individual macros for the day.

96. Protein bars (check sugar content)

Ingredient:

Protein Bars for Carb Cycling

When selecting protein bars for a carb cycling diet, it's important to check the nutrition label and choose bars that fit your macronutrient needs for that day.

Look for protein bars that:

• Have 15•20g of protein per serving
• Have 20•30g of carbs per serving, depending on your carb cycling needs
• Have minimal added sugars (aim for under 10g per serving)
• Are made with whole, nutrient•dense ingredients like nuts, seeds, oats, etc.

Some good options include:

• Quest Nutrition Protein Bars
• RxBar Protein Bars
• Evo Hemp Protein Bars
• Bulletproof Collagen Protein Bars

Avoid protein bars that are high in sugar, have a long list of artificial ingredients, or are very high in calories. These may not fit well into a balanced carb cycling plan.

Remember to adjust the portion size of the protein bar to match your individual macros for that day. A half or whole bar may be appropriate depending on your needs.

Pairing the protein bar with a piece of fruit or a small serving of nuts can also make for a more balanced snack on higher carb days.

97. Baked kale chips

Ingredient:

- 1 bunch kale, washed and dried thoroughly
- 1 tbsp olive oil
- 1/4 tsp sea salt

Instructions:

1. Preheat the oven to 325°F. Line a large baking sheet with parchment paper.

2. Tear the kale leaves into bite•sized pieces, discarding any thick stems. Place the kale in a large bowl.

3. Drizzle the olive oil over the kale and use your hands to massage the oil into the leaves, making sure they are all lightly coated.

4. Sprinkle the sea salt over the kale and toss to distribute evenly.

5. Arrange the kale leaves in a single layer on the prepared baking sheet, making sure they are not overlapping.

6. Bake for 12•15 minutes, flipping the kale halfway through, until the leaves are crispy.

7. Remove the kale chips from the oven and let cool completely before serving.

Nutrition Info (per serving, about 1 cup):
- Calories: 50
- Carbs: 5g
- Protein: 2g
- Fat: 3g
- Fiber: 2g

These baked kale chips make a great low•carb, high•fiber snack option for a carb cycling diet plan. The crunchy texture and salty flavor satisfy cravings while providing minimal carbs. Adjust the portion size as needed to fit your individual macros for the day.

98. Rice crackers with guacamole

Ingredient:

- 8•10 whole grain rice crackers
- 1 ripe avocado, mashed
- 1 tbsp diced tomato
- 1 tbsp diced onion
- 1 tsp lime juice
- 1/4 tsp sea salt
- 1/4 tsp ground cumin

Instructions:

1. In a small bowl, mash the avocado with a fork until smooth.

2. Stir in the diced tomato, onion, lime juice, sea salt, and cumin. Mix well to combine.

3. Spread the guacamole evenly over the rice crackers.

4. Serve immediately.

Nutrition Info (per serving, 2 crackers with guacamole):
- Calories: 150
- Carbs: 15g
- Protein: 3g
- Fat: 9g
- Fiber: 4g

This rice cracker and guacamole snack makes a great option for a lower carb day on a carb cycling plan. The rice crackers provide complex carbs, while the avocado in the guacamole adds healthy fats and fiber to keep you feeling full. Adjust the portion size as needed to fit your individual macros for the day.

99. Oatmeal with berries

Ingredient:

- 1/2 cup old•fashioned rolled oats
- 1 cup unsweetened almond milk (or milk of choice)
- 1/2 cup fresh or frozen berries (such as blueberries, raspberries, or strawberries)
- 1 tsp honey (optional)
- 1 tbsp chopped nuts or seeds (such as almonds, walnuts, or chia seeds)

Instructions:

1. In a small saucepan, combine the rolled oats and almond milk. Bring to a simmer over medium heat, stirring occasionally.

2. Reduce heat to low and continue cooking for 5•7 minutes, stirring frequently, until the oats have reached your desired consistency.

3. Remove the oatmeal from heat and stir in the berries. If using, drizzle the honey over the top.

4. Transfer the oatmeal to a bowl and top with the chopped nuts or seeds.

Nutrition Info (per serving):
- Calories: 300
- Carbs: 40g
- Protein: 10g
- Fat: 12g
- Fiber: 8g

This oatmeal with berries makes a great option for a higher carb day on a carb cycling plan. The oats provide complex carbs, while the berries add natural sweetness and antioxidants. The nuts or seeds add healthy fats and extra fiber. Adjust the portion size as needed to fit your individual macros for the day.

100. *Chocolate avocado mousse*

Ingredient:

- 1 ripe avocado, pitted and flesh scooped out
- 1/4 cup unsweetened cocoa powder
- 2 tbsp honey or maple syrup
- 1/4 cup unsweetened almond milk
- 1 tsp vanilla extract
- Pinch of sea salt

Instructions:

1. In a food processor or high•powered blender, combine the avocado, cocoa powder, honey/maple syrup, almond milk, vanilla, and sea salt. Blend until smooth and creamy, scraping down the sides as needed.

2. Taste and adjust sweetener as desired. The avocado provides a rich, creamy texture.

3. Transfer the chocolate mousse to individual serving dishes or ramekins. Refrigerate for at least 30 minutes before serving.

4. Top with fresh berries, chopped nuts, or a light dusting of cocoa powder before serving, if desired.

Nutrition Info (per serving, 1/2 cup):
- Calories: 150
- Carbs: 15g
- Protein: 3g
- Fat: 10g
- Fiber: 6g

This chocolate avocado mousse makes a great low•carb, high•fat dessert option for a carb cycling diet plan. The healthy fats from the avocado and minimal added sweetener make it a nutritious treat. Adjust the portion size as needed to fit your individual macros for the day.

101. Mango sorbet

Ingredient:

- 2 cups frozen mango chunks
- 1/4 cup unsweetened almond milk
- 1 tbsp honey (optional)
- 1 tsp lime juice

Instructions:

1. In a high•powered blender or food processor, combine the frozen mango chunks, almond milk, honey (if using), and lime juice.

2. Blend on high speed, stopping to scrape down the sides as needed, until the mixture is smooth and creamy, resembling a sorbet texture.

3. Serve the mango sorbet immediately for a soft, scoopable consistency. For a firmer texture, transfer the sorbet to a freezer•safe container and freeze for 1•2 hours before serving.

Nutrition Info (per serving, 1/2 cup):
- Calories: 100
- Carbs: 20g
- Protein: 1g
- Fat: 1g
- Fiber: 2g

This mango sorbet makes a great option for a higher carb day on a carb cycling plan. The natural sweetness from the mango provides carbs, while the minimal added honey and almond milk keep it light and refreshing. Adjust the portion size as needed to fit your individual macros for the day.

102. Banana smoothie with oats

Ingredient:

- 1 ripe banana, frozen
- 1/2 cup unsweetened almond milk
- 1/4 cup old•fashioned rolled oats
- 1 tbsp peanut butter (or other nut butter)
- 1 tsp honey (optional)
- 1/2 tsp vanilla extract
- Pinch of cinnamon

Instructions:

1. In a high•powered blender, combine the frozen banana, almond milk, rolled oats, peanut butter, honey (if using), vanilla, and cinnamon.

2. Blend on high speed until the mixture is smooth and creamy.

3. Pour the banana smoothie into a glass and enjoy immediately.

Nutrition Info (per serving):
- Calories: 300
- Carbs: 40g
- Protein: 10g
- Fat: 12g
- Fiber: 6g

This banana smoothie with oats makes a great option for a higher carb day on a carb cycling plan. The banana and oats provide complex carbs, while the peanut butter adds healthy fats and protein to keep you feeling full. Adjust the portion size as needed to fit your individual macros for the day.

103. Almond flour muffins

Ingredient:

- 2 cups almond flour
- 1/4 cup coconut flour
- 1 tsp baking powder
- 1/4 tsp sea salt
- 3 large eggs
- 1/4 cup unsweetened almond milk
- 2 tbsp melted coconut oil
- 2 tbsp honey or maple syrup
- 1 tsp vanilla extract

Instructions:

1. Preheat the oven to 350°F. Grease a 12•cup muffin tin or line with paper liners.

2. In a medium bowl, whisk together the almond flour, coconut flour, baking powder, and sea salt.

3. In a separate bowl, beat the eggs. Then stir in the almond milk, melted coconut oil, honey/maple syrup, and vanilla.

4. Pour the wet ingredients into the dry ingredients and mix just until combined, being careful not to overmix.

5. Divide the batter evenly among the prepared muffin cups, filling them about 3/4 full.

6. Bake for 18•22 minutes, until a toothpick inserted in the center comes out clean.

7. Allow the muffins to cool in the tin for 5 minutes before transferring to a wire rack.

Nutrition Info (per muffin):
- Calories: 150
- Carbs: 8g
- Protein: 5g
- Fat: 12g
- Fiber: 3g

These almond flour muffins make a great low•carb option for a carb cycling diet plan. The almond and coconut flours provide healthy fats and minimal carbs. Adjust the portion size as needed to fit your individual macros for the day.

104. Quinoa energy bites

Ingredient:

- 1 cup cooked quinoa, cooled
- 1/2 cup almond butter
- 1/4 cup honey
- 1/4 cup unsweetened shredded coconut
- 2 tbsp chia seeds
- 1 tsp vanilla extract
- Pinch of sea salt

Instructions:

1. In a medium bowl, combine the cooked quinoa, almond butter, honey, shredded coconut, chia seeds, vanilla, and sea salt. Mix well until fully incorporated.

2. Using a tablespoon or small cookie scoop, form the mixture into bite•sized balls and place them on a parchment•lined baking sheet.

3. Refrigerate the energy bites for at least 30 minutes to allow them to firm up.

4. Store the quinoa energy bites in an airtight container in the refrigerator for up to 1 week.

Nutrition Info (per serving, 1 energy bite):
- Calories: 100
- Carbs: 10g
- Protein: 3g
- Fat: 6g
- Fiber: 2g

These quinoa energy bites make a great portable snack option for a carb cycling diet plan. The quinoa provides complex carbs, while the almond butter and chia seeds add healthy fats and protein. Adjust the portion size as needed to fit your individual macros for the day.

105. Frozen grapes

Ingredient:
• 1 lb seedless grapes, washed and dried

Instructions:

1. Spread the grapes in a single layer on a baking sheet or plate.

2. Place the baking sheet or plate in the freezer and freeze the grapes for at least 2 hours, or until completely frozen.

3. Once frozen, transfer the grapes to an airtight container or resealable plastic bag. Store in the freezer for up to 3 months.

Nutrition Info (per 1/2 cup serving):
• Calories: 60
• Carbs: 15g
• Protein: 1g
• Fat: 0g
• Fiber: 1g

Frozen grapes make a great low•calorie, high•carb snack option for a carb cycling diet plan. The natural sweetness of the grapes provides a refreshing treat, while the freezing process gives them a fun, icy texture.

Adjust the portion size as needed to fit your individual carb macros for the day. Frozen grapes can be enjoyed on their own or paired with a small serving of nuts or a protein source for a more balanced snack.

The simplicity and convenience of this recipe makes it an easy go•to option to have on hand during your carb cycling journey.

106. Cucumber slices with tzatziki

Ingredient:

- 1 English cucumber, sliced into rounds
- 1 cup plain Greek yogurt
- 1 tbsp lemon juice
- 1 garlic clove, minced
- 1 tbsp chopped fresh dill
- 1/4 tsp sea salt
- 1/4 tsp ground black pepper

Instructions:

1. In a medium bowl, combine the Greek yogurt, lemon juice, garlic, dill, salt, and pepper. Stir until well mixed.

2. Arrange the cucumber slices on a serving platter or plate.

3. Spoon the tzatziki sauce over the cucumber slices, making sure to coat them evenly.

4. Serve immediately or refrigerate until ready to serve.

Nutrition Info (per serving, 4•5 cucumber slices with 2 tbsp tzatziki):
- Calories: 80
- Carbs: 6g
- Protein: 6g
- Fat: 3g
- Fiber: 1g

This cucumber and tzatziki snack makes a great option for a lower carb day on a carb cycling plan. The cucumber provides a crunchy, hydrating base, while the tzatziki sauce adds protein and healthy fats from the Greek yogurt. Adjust the portion size as needed to fit your individual macros for the day.

107. Pistachios

Ingredient:

- 4 salmon fillets (about 6 oz each)
- 1 cup shelled pistachios, finely chopped
- 2 tbsp panko breadcrumbs
- 2 tbsp grated Parmesan cheese
- 1 tsp lemon zest
- 1/4 tsp salt
- 1/4 tsp black pepper
- 2 tbsp olive oil

Instructions:

1. Preheat oven to 400°F. Line a baking sheet with parchment paper.

2. In a shallow bowl, mix together the chopped pistachios, panko, Parmesan, lemon zest, salt and pepper.

3. Brush the top of each salmon fillet lightly with olive oil.

4. Press the pistachio mixture firmly onto the top of each salmon fillet, coating completely.

5. Place the salmon fillets, pistachio side up, on the prepared baking sheet.

6. Bake for 12•15 minutes, until the salmon is cooked through and the pistachio crust is golden brown.

7. Serve the pistachio crusted salmon immediately. Enjoy!

The crunchy pistachio topping adds a wonderful nutty flavor and texture to the tender salmon.

108. Sliced turkey with mustard

Ingredient:

- 8 oz sliced turkey breast
- 1 tbsp Dijon mustard
- 1 tsp olive oil
- 1/4 tsp dried thyme
- Salt and pepper to taste

Instructions:

1. In a small bowl, mix together the Dijon mustard, olive oil, and dried thyme. Season with a pinch of salt and pepper.

2. Lay the sliced turkey breast in a single layer on a plate or baking sheet.

3. Spoon the mustard mixture over the turkey slices and use the back of a spoon to spread it evenly over the top.

4. Let the turkey sit for 5•10 minutes to allow the flavors to meld.

5. Serve the sliced turkey with mustard as part of a carb cycling meal. It pairs well with steamed vegetables, a small portion of brown rice or quinoa, or a side salad.

This recipe is low in carbs and high in protein, making it a great option for a lower carb day on a carb cycling diet plan. The mustard adds flavor without adding many calories or carbs. Feel free to adjust the amount of mustard to your taste preference.

109. Pita chips with salsa

Ingredient:
- 4 whole wheat pita breads, cut into triangles
- 1 tbsp olive oil
- 1/2 tsp garlic powder
- 1/4 tsp salt

For the Salsa:
- 1 cup diced tomatoes
- 1/4 cup diced onion
- 2 tbsp chopped cilantro
- 1 tbsp lime juice
- 1/4 tsp cumin
- 1/4 tsp chili powder
- Salt and pepper to taste

Instructions:

1. Preheat oven to 400°F. Line a baking sheet with parchment paper.

2. In a large bowl, toss the pita triangles with the olive oil, garlic powder and salt until evenly coated.

3. Spread the pita triangles in a single layer on the prepared baking sheet.

4. Bake for 8•10 minutes, flipping halfway, until lightly golden and crispy.

5. Meanwhile, in a medium bowl, mix together all the salsa ingredients. Season with salt and pepper to taste.

6. Serve the homemade pita chips warm with the fresh salsa on the side.

This makes a great snack or appetizer for a carb cycling diet plan. The pita chips are a complex carb source, while the salsa provides fiber, vitamins and antioxidants without many carbs. Adjust portion sizes as needed for your carb cycling macros.

110. Cheese cubes

Ingredient:

• 8 oz block of cheddar cheese, cut into 1•inch cubes
• Optional seasonings: garlic powder, paprika, dried herbs

Instructions:

1. Cut the block of cheddar cheese into 1•inch cubes.

2. If desired, you can season the cheese cubes with a light sprinkle of garlic powder, paprika, dried oregano, or other dried herbs. This adds extra flavor.

3. Arrange the cheese cubes on a plate or in a container.

4. Serve the cheese cubes as a snack or pair them with other low•carb items like sliced turkey, nuts, or fresh vegetables.

The cheese cubes provide a good source of protein and healthy fats without any carbs, making them an ideal snack for a carb cycling diet plan. They can be enjoyed on lower carb days.

Some tips:
• Choose a full•fat cheddar or other hard cheese for the most nutrients.
• Avoid pre•shredded cheese, as it often contains added starches.
• Portion the cheese cubes into 1•2 oz servings to keep the calories in check.

Congratulations on reaching the end of ***Carb Cycling Diet Plan & Cookbook: Recipes for Weight Loss, Muscle Building, Effective Exercise Plans with 60-Day Meal Plans and 110 Delicious Recipes!*** By now, you have delved into the principles of carb cycling, explored effective exercise plans, and discovered a variety of delicious recipes to support your health and fitness goals.

Recap and Reflection

Throughout this book, we have provided you with a comprehensive guide to carb cycling, focusing on the balance of high-carb and low-carb days to optimize your metabolism and energy levels. We've highlighted:

- ***The Basics of Carb Cycling:*** Understanding the science behind carb cycling and how it can aid in weight loss and muscle building.

- ***Effective Exercise Plans:*** Incorporating the right mix of cardio and strength training to complement your dietary efforts.

- ***60-Day Meal Plans:*** Structured meal plans to guide you through your first two months, making it easier to stay on track.

- ***110 Nutritious Recipes:*** A diverse array of recipes that are both delicious and aligned with your carb cycling goals.

Moving Forward

As you continue on your health and fitness journey, remember that consistency and patience are key. The habits you've developed and the knowledge you've gained from this book will serve as a strong foundation for ongoing success. Here are a few tips to keep in mind:

- ***Listen to Your Body:*** Pay attention to how your body responds to different foods and exercise routines, and adjust as needed.

- ***Stay Flexible:*** Life is unpredictable, and it's okay to adapt your plan when necessary. The goal is sustainable progress, not perfection.

- ***Celebrate Your Successes:*** No matter how small, every step forward is a victory. Celebrate your achievements and use them as motivation to keep going.

Thank you for choosing this book as your guide. We wish you continued success, happiness, and health.